THE COMPREHENSIVE DIABETES FOOD LIST AND MEAL PLAN

REVERSE DIABETES WITH THE KIND OF FOOD YOU CHOOSE AND BE HEALTHY

TONY B. SCOTT

Copyright Page

Copyright © 2023 by TONY B. SCOTT

This nonfiction book is a work of [insert genre or subject]. The information and opinions presented in this book are solely those of the author and do not necessarily reflect the views or endorsements of any individuals, organizations, or institutions mentioned within.

Disclaimer: The information presented in this book is for informational purposes only. The author and publisher have made efforts to ensure the accuracy and completeness of the contents, but they make no warranties or representations, either expressed or implied, with respect to the accuracy, completeness, or suitability of the information provided. The author and publisher disclaim any liability for any errors, omissions, or damages arising from the use of this book or any materials contained within it.

This copyright page applies to the printed version of the book. Please refer to the appropriate ebook edition for the applicable copyright page.

Table of content

Introduction To "The Comprehensive Diabetes Food List and Meal Plan"

Greetings! Welcome to the introduction of the book "Comprehensive Diabetes Food List and Meal Plan." In this insightful and informative guide, we dive deep into the world of diabetes management through nutrition. This book aims to be a comprehensive resource, providing you with an extensive food list and a well-designed meal plan specifically tailored for individuals living with diabetes.

Living with diabetes can present various challenges, and one crucial aspect of managing the condition is maintaining a healthy and balanced diet. However, navigating the countless food options and deciphering their impact on blood sugar levels can be overwhelming. That's where this book comes to your aid.

Our team of experts has meticulously crafted a food list that categorizes various types of food based on their impact on blood sugar levels. This carefully curated list offers you a comprehensive understanding of which foods to include, limit, or avoid to effectively manage your blood sugar levels.

Yet, we understand that knowledge alone is not enough. That's why this book also provides you with a well-structured meal plan. This meal plan not only incorporates the recommended foods from the comprehensive list but also offers a diverse range of options to ensure your meals are both nutritious and enjoyable. With this guide, you'll discover a wealth of delicious meal ideas that align with your dietary needs and diabetes management goals.

Furthermore, our meal plan is designed to not only regulate blood sugar levels but also support weight management and promote overall health. We understand the importance of maintaining a healthy weight in diabetes management and have created a meal plan that takes this into consideration. By following this plan, you'll not only be better equipped to manage your blood sugar levels but also maintain a healthy weight and improve your overall well-being.

Whether you're new to diabetes management or a seasoned veteran, this book provides you with an invaluable resource to enhance your dietary choices and improve your health. The detailed food list and meal plan will empower you to take control of your diabetes management, making informed decisions about your food consumption and ultimately leading to a happier and healthier lifestyle.

So, join us on this journey towards better diabetes management through nutrition. With the "Comprehensive Diabetes Food List and Meal Plan" book as your guide, you'll gain the knowledge and tools necessary to make proactive choices that positively impact your diabetes management and overall well-being.

Chapter 1. Introduction to Diabetes

Welcome to this comprehensive introductory note about diabetes. Whether you are newly diagnosed or seeking to expand your knowledge on this chronic condition, we are here to provide you with a comprehensive overview that will help you understand the ins and outs of diabetics,

Greetings and welcome to our thorough introduction to diabetes. We are here to give you a thorough overview that will help you comprehend the ins and outs of diabetes, regardless of whether you are looking to learn more about this chronic condition or have just received your diagnosis.

Millions of individuals throughout the world suffer with diabetes, a chronic medical condition. It happens when the body has trouble successfully controlling blood sugar levels. If left unchecked, this inability to keep blood sugar levels steady can have detrimental repercussions on the body's systems and organs.

The two primary form of diabetes are: type 1 and type 2. One form of diabetes is autoimmune. While type 2 diabetes can sometimes be managed with lifestyle changes alone, medications or insulin may also be prescribed to help control blood sugar levels.

Beyond type 1 and type 2 diabetes, there are other forms of diabetes, such as gestational diabetes, which occurs during pregnancy, and prediabetes, where individuals have higher than normal blood sugar levels but not yet in the diabetic range. It is important to note that both prediabetes and gestational diabetes can increase the risk of developing type 2 diabetes later in life.

The impact of diabetes goes beyond just blood sugar regulation. It can affect various systems in the body, including the cardiovascular system, kidneys, eyes, and nerves. Uncontrolled diabetes can lead to complications such as heart disease, stroke, kidney disease, vision problems, and nerve damage.

The good news is that diabetes can be effectively managed with the right knowledge, lifestyle modifications, and appropriate medical care. A key component of diabetes management revolves around maintaining a healthy diet, engaging in regular exercise, monitoring blood sugar levels, taking prescribed medications or insulin, and regularly visiting healthcare professionals.

In this note, we will explore various aspects of diabetes management, including dietary considerations, exercise recommendations, medication options, and tips for preventing complications. We will provide you with evidence-based information, practical tips, and valuable insights to support you in your journey towards living a fulfilling and healthy life with diabetes.

We understand that managing diabetes can be challenging, but rest assured, you are not alone. By equipping yourself with knowledge and adopting a proactive approach to your health, you can take control of your diabetes and lead a vibrant and fulfilling life.

So, let's embark on this informative journey together as we delve into the complexities of diabetes, demystify its management, and empower you with the tools to thrive while living with this chronic condition.
Wishing you health and vitality.

Understanding Diabetes

Welcome to this comprehensive note on understanding diabetes. In this guide, we will delve into the intricacies of diabetes, providing you with a thorough understanding of the condition and its impact on the body. Whether you have recently been diagnosed with diabetes, are caring for someone with the condition, or simply want to expand your knowledge, this note will serve as a valuable resource.

Diabetes is a chronic health condition that affects the body's ability to regulate blood sugar levels. It occurs when the pancreas either does not produce enough insulin (a hormone responsible for regulating blood sugar) or when the body cannot effectively use the insulin it produces. This results in elevated blood sugar levels, also known as hyperglycemia.

Diabetes comes in various forms, the most prevalent being type 1 and type 2. An autoimmune condition known as type 1 diabetes occurs when the immune system unintentionally targets and kills the pancreatic cells that produce insulin. This requires individuals with type 1 diabetes to rely on insulin injections or the use of an insulin pump to manage their blood sugar levels effectively.

Type 2 diabetes, on the other hand, is characterized by insulin resistance or the body's reduced ability to use insulin. It is often associated with lifestyle factors such as poor diet, lack of physical activity, and obesity. Type 2 diabetes develops gradually over time and may not exhibit noticeable symptoms in the early stages. Lifestyle changes, such as healthy eating, regular physical activity, and weight management, are essential for managing type 2 diabetes. In some cases, oral medications or insulin therapy may also be prescribed.

Another type of diabetes that develops during pregnancy is called gestational diabetes. It affects some women who have never had diabetes before and usually resolves after giving birth. However, women with gestational diabetes have an increased risk of developing type 2 diabetes later in life.

Understanding diabetes extends beyond recognizing the different types. It is vital to grasp its impact on various organs and systems in the body. Uncontrolled diabetes can lead to long-term complications affecting the cardiovascular system, kidneys, eyes, nerves, and other organs. These complications include heart disease, stroke, kidney disease, diabetic retinopathy, neuropathy, and foot ulcers. Managing diabetes effectively is crucial to preventing or minimizing the risk of these complications.

Key components of diabetes management include maintaining a healthy diet, engaging in regular physical activity, monitoring blood sugar levels, taking prescribed medications or insulin, and attending regular check-ups with healthcare professionals. These measures help to control blood sugar levels, reduce the risk of complications, and promote overall well-being.

Education and awareness are fundamental to living well with diabetes. Through this note, we aim to provide you with an in-depth understanding of the condition, its causes, risk factors, symptoms, diagnosis, and treatment options. We will explore strategies for managing diabetes effectively, including meal planning, exercise recommendations, blood sugar monitoring, and stress management.

You are not alone on this journey. Diabetes support networks, online communities, and healthcare professionals can provide valuable guidance and assistance. By equipping yourself with knowledge, adopting a positive mindset, and making informed decisions about your health, you can lead a fulfilling and empowered life with diabetes.

Remember, successful diabetes management requires proactive self-care, ongoing education, and collaboration with healthcare providers. Together, we can demystify diabetes and empower you to take control of your health.

Types of Diabetes

Diabetes is a complex condition that encompasses different types, each with its unique characteristics. Here's a comprehensive overview of the main types of diabetes:

1. **Type 1 Diabetes**: Type 1 diabetes, often diagnosed in childhood or adolescence, is an autoimmune disease. Little to no insulin is produced when the immune system unintentionally targets and kills the pancreatic cells that produce insulin. People with type 1 diabetes require lifelong insulin injections or the use of an insulin pump to regulate their blood sugar levels.

2. **Type 2 Diabetes**: Type 2 diabetes is the most common form, accounting for the

majority of diabetes cases. It typically develops later in life but can occur at any age. In type 2 diabetes, the body becomes resistant to insulin or fails to use it effectively. Its development is aided by lifestyle factors like obesity, sedentary behavior, and poor diet. Initially, the recommendations are for weight management, lifestyle changes, and oral medications; however, some patients may also require insulin therapy.

3. Gestational Diabetes: Some women who have never had diabetes before develop gestational diabetes during pregnancy. Elevated blood sugar levels during pregnancy can be caused by hormonal changes and insulin resistance.

Gestational diabetes usually resolves after childbirth, but it increases the risk of type

2 diabetes later in life for both the mother and the child.

4. Prediabetes: Prediabetes is a condition where blood sugar levels are higher than normal but not yet at the level of diabetes. It serves as a warning sign that one is at risk of developing type 2 diabetes if lifestyle changes are not made. With early intervention and lifestyle modifications such as weight loss, healthy eating, and regular physical activity, the progression to type 2 diabetes can often be delayed or prevented.

5. Other Types: Less common types of diabetes include monogenic diabetes, which is caused by genetic mutations affecting insulin production, and secondary diabetes, resulting from other medical conditions or medications that interfere with insulin function.

Understanding the different types of diabetes allows individuals to navigate their condition and make informed decisions about their management plan. It is important to work closely with healthcare professionals to receive an accurate diagnosis, personalized treatment, and ongoing support for optimal diabetes care.

Remember, every individual's experience with diabetes is unique, and treatment approaches may vary. Stay informed, engage in self-care, and reach out to healthcare providers or diabetes support networks for guidance on managing your specific type of diabetes effectively.

To get a more in-depth understanding and tailored information about your specific diabetes type, consult with a healthcare professional.

Importance of a Comprehensive Diabetes Meal Plan

Today, I would like to highlight the importance of a comprehensive diabetes meal plan in managing diabetes effectively. A well-designed meal plan plays a crucial role in achieving optimal blood sugar control, maintaining a healthy weight, and promoting overall well-being for individuals living with diabetes.

When it comes to diabetes management, proper nutrition is essential. A comprehensive diabetes meal plan provides guidance on selecting the right foods, controlling portion sizes, and balancing macronutrients (carbohydrates, proteins, and fats) to help manage blood sugar levels effectively.

Let's delve into the key reasons why a comprehensive diabetes meal plan is of utmost importance:

1. **Blood Sugar Control**: Managing blood sugar levels is a primary goal of diabetes management. A diabetes meal plan allows you to choose foods that have a minimal impact on blood sugar levels, reducing the risk of blood sugar spikes and crashes. By selecting the right combination of carbohydrates, proteins, and fats and

spreading your meals and snacks evenly throughout the day, you can regulate blood sugar levels and maintain stability.

2. Nutritional Balance: A comprehensive diabetes meal plan ensures that your nutritional needs are met while managing your condition. It emphasizes the importance of incorporating a wide variety of nutrient-dense foods, such as fruits, vegetables, whole grains, lean proteins, and healthy fats. This balance helps provide essential vitamins, minerals, fiber, and antioxidants that support overall health and reduce the risk of complications associated with diabetes.

3. Weight Management: It's critical for people with diabetes to reach and stay at a healthy weight. A diabetes meal plan can be tailored to support weight management goals, whether it involves weight loss or weight maintenance. By providing portion control guidance, promoting healthier food choices, and encouraging mindful eating practices, a meal plan can help you reach and sustain a healthy weight, which in turn contributes to better blood sugar control and overall well-being.

4. Personalization and Flexibility: Every person's diabetes management needs are unique. A comprehensive diabetes meal plan takes into account your personal preferences, cultural background, lifestyle, and existing health conditions. It allows for customization and flexibility to meet your specific dietary requirements, making it more convenient, enjoyable, and sustainable. Whether you adhere to a vegetarian or Mediterranean-style diet, have food allergies or sensitivities, or need to accommodate specific cultural or religious dietary practices, a meal plan can be adapted to suit your needs.

5. Long-Term Success: Diabetes is a chronic condition that requires long-term management. Having a comprehensive meal plan provides structure and support for making healthier food choices consistently. It helps create sustainable habits and reduces the likelihood of making impulsive or unhealthy food choices that can negatively impact blood sugar control. Over time, embracing a well-designed meal plan can become second nature, empowering you to take charge of your diabetes management in the long term.

Remember, a comprehensive diabetes meal plan is just one component of overall diabetes management. It is crucial to work alongside healthcare professionals, such as registered dietitians or certified diabetes educators, to design a meal plan that fits your specific needs and aligns with your overall treatment plan.

By adopting a comprehensive diabetes meal plan, you can take proactive steps towards better blood sugar control, improved nutrition, weight management, and overall well-being. Embrace the power of food and nourish your body with the right choices to thrive with diabetes.

Chapter 2. Basics of Diabetes Management

Today, let's dive into the basics of diabetes management. Whether you have recently been diagnosed with diabetes or are looking for a refresher, understanding the fundamental principles of effective diabetes management is essential for achieving optimal health and well-being. Here, we will explore key areas of focus in diabetes management to help you navigate this condition successfully.

1. **Blood Sugar Monitoring**: Regularly monitoring blood sugar levels is crucial in diabetes management. This involves using a blood glucose meter to measure your blood sugar levels at specific times throughout the day. Keeping track of your

blood sugar levels helps you understand how different foods, activities, medications, and stress levels impact your blood sugar, allowing you to make necessary adjustments to your diabetes management plan.

2. Healthy Eating: Proper nutrition is a cornerstone of diabetes management. Following a healthy eating plan that focuses on balanced meals and portion control is vital. Emphasize consuming nutrient-dense, whole foods such as fruits, vegetables, whole grains, lean proteins, and healthy fats while limiting processed foods, sugary beverages, and foods high in saturated or trans fats. Consulting with a registered dietitian or certified diabetes educator can help you create an individualized meal plan that suits your dietary preferences and diabetes management goals.

3. Regular Physical Activity: Engaging in regular physical activity is beneficial for managing blood sugar levels, enhancing insulin sensitivity, managing weight, and improving overall cardiovascular health. Aim for at least 150 minutes of moderate-intensity aerobic exercise, such as brisk walking, swimming, or cycling, spread throughout the week. To increase muscle and speed up your metabolism, add strength training exercises to your routine two or more days a week. Always consult with your healthcare team before starting any exercise program and tailor activities to your abilities and fitness level.

4. Medication Management: Depending on the type of diabetes you have, you may need to take oral medications or insulin to help control blood sugar levels. It is essential to take your prescribed medications as directed, follow proper injection techniques if using insulin, and communicate any concerns or side effects to your healthcare provider. Medication management includes timing medication doses appropriately, understanding potential interactions with food or other medications, and regularly checking in with your healthcare team to assess the effectiveness of your current treatment plan.

5. **Stress Management**: Stress can affect blood sugar levels and overall well-being. Finding healthy ways to manage stress, such as practicing mindfulness, engaging in relaxation techniques (e.g., deep breathing exercises, yoga, or meditation),

or pursuing hobbies and activities you enjoy, can positively impact your diabetes management. Seek support from friends, family, or mental health professionals when needed to prioritize your emotional well-being.

6. Regular Medical Check-ups: Schedule regular visits with your healthcare team to monitor your diabetes management progress, address any concerns or questions, and assess your overall health. These check-ups may include measurements of blood pressure, weight, cholesterol levels, kidney function tests, and eye exams. Regular dental and foot examinations are also important to identify and address any potential complications associated with diabetes.

Remember, effectively managing diabetes requires an individualized approach tailored to your specific needs. Working closely with your healthcare team, which may include endocrinologists, registered dietitians, certified diabetes educators, nurses, and other specialists, can provide the guidance and support necessary to optimize your diabetes management plan.

By implementing these fundamental principles of diabetes management into your daily routine, you can take control of your health, reduce the risk of complications, and lead a fulfilling life with diabetes. Stay informed, engaged, and proactive in managing your diabetes, and remember that with the right support, education, and self-care, you can thrive while managing this chronic condition.

Blood Sugar Control and Monitoring

Maintaining proper blood sugar control is crucial for individuals with diabetes, as well as those at risk of developing the condition. Blood sugar, also known as blood glucose, refers to the amount of sugar present in your blood. It is regulated by hormone insulin, produced by the pancreas. Failure to control blood sugar levels can lead to various complications such as heart disease, kidney damage, and nerve damage. This note will provide a comprehensive overview of blood sugar control and monitoring, including tips for managing blood sugar levels effectively.

1. Importance of Blood Sugar Control:
Maintaining optimal blood sugar levels is essential for overall health and

well-being. Uncontrolled blood sugar can lead to both short-term and long-term complications. Short-term complications include hyperglycemia (high blood sugar) and hypoglycemia (low blood sugar), whereas long-term complications include cardiovascular disease, kidney disease, nerve damage, and eye damage. By monitoring and managing blood sugar levels, individuals can reduce the risk of these complications and maintain better overall health.

2. Self-Monitoring of Blood Sugar:
Self-monitoring of blood sugar involves regularly checking glucose levels using blood glucose meters or continuous glucose monitoring (CGM) systems. The frequency of monitoring can vary depending on individual needs, but it is typically recommended to test at least

several times a day. Self-monitoring provides valuable information about blood sugar patterns, helping individuals make appropriate lifestyle and medication adjustments. It also allows for early detection of high or low blood sugar episodes, enabling prompt action to prevent complications.

3. Healthy Lifestyle Strategies for Blood Sugar Control:

a. Balanced Diet: Eating a balanced diet that includes a variety of whole grains, lean proteins, fruits, vegetables, and healthy fats is crucial for managing blood sugar levels. It's especially crucial to stay away from refined carbohydrates and sugary foods.

b. Regular Exercise: Engaging in regular physical activity can help improve insulin sensitivity and lower blood sugar levels. Aim for at least 150 minutes of moderate-intensity aerobic exercise per week, along with resistance training for muscle strength.

c. Medication Management: Individuals with diabetes may need to take medication, such as insulin or oral hypoglycemic agents, to control their blood sugar levels. Following prescribed medication regimens is vital for maintaining stable blood sugar control.

d. Stress Management: Stress can affect blood sugar levels, so practicing stress reduction techniques like mindfulness, meditation, and relaxation exercises can be beneficial.

e. Sufficient Sleep: Lack of sleep can disrupt blood sugar levels and insulin sensitivity. 7-9 hours of well-rested sleep each night is the goal.

f. Limit Alcohol Consumption: Alcohol can cause fluctuations in blood sugar levels and affect the liver's ability to regulate blood sugar. Moderation is key; men should not exceed two drinks per day, and women should limit alcohol intake to one drink per day.

4. Treatment Options for Blood Sugar Control:

Depending on the individual's condition, various treatment options may be recommended, including:

a. Insulin Therapy: This involves using injectable insulin to maintain normal blood sugar levels. The dosage and administration frequency are determined based on the individual's needs.

b. Oral Medications: Non-insulin oral medications may be prescribed to improve blood sugar control. These medications can increase insulin sensitivity, decrease glucose production in the liver, or slow carbohydrate absorption.

c. Lifestyle Modifications: As mentioned earlier, adopting a healthy lifestyle with regular exercise and a balanced diet can significantly contribute to blood sugar control.

5. Regular Medical Check-ups:

Regular medical check-ups with healthcare professionals are essential for managing blood sugar levels effectively. These visits allow for comprehensive monitoring of blood sugar, evaluation of treatment effectiveness, adjustment of medication dosages, and screening for any complications associated with diabetes.

Conclusion:

Maintaining blood sugar control is crucial for individuals with diabetes and those at risk of developing the condition. By regularly monitoring blood glucose levels, adopting a healthy lifestyle, following prescribed medication regimens, and seeking regular medical check-ups, individuals can effectively control their blood sugar levels and reduce the risk of complications. It is advised to work closely with healthcare professionals to develop an individualized plan for blood sugar control based on specific needs and circumstances.

Role of Diet in Diabetes

Diet plays a fundamental role in managing diabetes. Proper nutrition is essential for maintaining stable blood sugar levels, preventing complications, and promoting overall health and well-being. This comprehensive note will outline the key aspects of a diabetes-friendly diet, including recommended food choices, portion control, meal planning, and important considerations for managing blood sugar levels effectively.

1. Importance of Diet in Diabetes Management:

Dietary choices have a direct impact on blood sugar levels in individuals with diabetes. By making healthy food choices, managing portion sizes, and understanding the glycemic index of foods (which measures how quickly they raise blood sugar levels), individuals can:

a. Achieve and maintain target blood glucose levels

b. Manage weight effectively

c. Reduce the risk of cardiovascular complications

d. Prevent or delay the onset of complications associated with diabetes

2. Key Components of a Diabetes-Friendly Diet:

a. Carbohydrates: Carbohydrates have the most significant impact on blood sugar levels. It is important to choose healthy, low glycemic index carbohydrates, such as whole grains, legumes, fruits, and vegetables. Avoid or minimize high glycemic index foods like white bread, sugary snacks, and refined grains.

b. Proteins: Including lean proteins, such as poultry, fish, tofu, lentils, and beans, in meals can help control blood sugar levels and promote satiety. A balanced diet of protein should be consumed throughout the day.

c. Fats: Focus on consuming healthy fats like avocados, nuts, seeds, and olive oil while limiting saturated and trans fats. These healthier fats can help improve heart health and aid in blood sugar control.

d. Fiber: High-fiber foods, including whole grains, fruits, vegetables, and legumes, can slow down the absorption of carbohydrates, improve blood sugar control, and support overall digestive health.

e. Portion Control: Controlling portion sizes is essential in managing blood sugar levels. Monitoring the quantity of carbohydrates, proteins, and fats consumed can help prevent blood sugar spikes. Working with a registered dietitian can provide guidance on appropriate serving sizes for various foods.

3. Meal Planning for Diabetes:

a. Balanced Meals: Aim for balanced meals that include a variety of food groups. Fill half of your plate with non-starchy vegetables, one-fourth with lean proteins, and one-fourth with whole grains or starchy vegetables.

b. Snacking: Choose healthy, low-glycemic snacks when needed to prevent blood sugar fluctuations between meals. Examples include fresh fruit, raw vegetables with hummus, or a handful of nuts.

c. Regular Meal Timing: Consistency in meal timing can help regulate blood sugar levels. Aim for regular meal intervals, and if needed, add snacks to prevent prolonged hunger or hypoglycemia.

d. Glycemic Load Consideration: Along with the glycemic index, consider the glycemic load of a meal, which takes into account both the carbohydrate content and the amount consumed. Balancing low glycemic load foods with higher glycemic load foods helps maintain blood sugar control.

4. Individualized Approach:

Dietary recommendations may vary depending on individual factors, such as age, weight, activity level, medications, and any existing health conditions. It is crucial for individuals with diabetes to work closely with a registered dietitian and healthcare team to develop a personalized meal plan based on their specific needs.

5. Regular Monitoring and Adjustment:
Monitoring blood sugar levels regularly, either through self-monitoring or continuous glucose monitoring, can help individuals understand how different foods affect their blood sugar levels. This information can guide adjustments to the diet, such as modifying portion sizes, meal composition, or timing.

Conclusion:

A well-planned and balanced diet is a cornerstone of diabetes management. By focusing on low glycemic index carbohydrates, lean proteins, healthy fats, and high-fiber foods, individuals with diabetes can achieve better blood sugar control, reduce the risk of complications, and promote overall health. It is essential to work closely with healthcare professionals, including registered dietitians, to develop an individualized meal plan that addresses specific needs and supports optimal diabetes management.

Benefits of a Comprehensive Meal Plan

A comprehensive meal plan refers to a well-structured and balanced approach to daily eating that incorporates various food groups, portion control, and nutrient considerations. Following a comprehensive meal plan offers numerous benefits for overall health, weight management, disease prevention, and overall well-being. This note will outline the advantages of adopting a comprehensive meal plan and how it can positively impact various aspects of an individual's life.

1. Optimal Nutrition:

A comprehensive meal plan ensures a well-rounded intake of essential nutrients, vitamins, and minerals required for optimal health. By incorporating a variety of food groups, including fruits, vegetables, lean proteins, whole grains, and healthy fats, individuals can meet their nutritional needs and maintain a balanced diet. This leads to improved overall nutrient intake, which supports proper physical and mental functioning.

2. Weight Management:

One of the key benefits of a comprehensive meal plan is its effectiveness in achieving and maintaining a healthy weight. By planning meals that are portion-controlled, based on individual needs and goals, individuals can better manage calorie intake. Additionally, a balanced meal plan comprised of nutrient-dense foods can provide satiety and prevent excessive snacking or overeating, supporting weight control efforts.

3. Blood Sugar Control:

A comprehensive meal plan is particularly beneficial for individuals with diabetes or those aiming to manage their blood sugar levels. By incorporating foods with a low glycemic index, balancing macronutrients, and controlling portion sizes, blood sugar levels can be better regulated. This leads to more stable energy levels throughout the day and helps prevent spikes and crashes in blood sugar, reducing the risk of complications associated with diabetes.

4. Heart Health:

Adopting a comprehensive meal plan that includes heart-healthy foods can significantly benefit cardiovascular health. By reducing the intake of saturated and trans fats, refined sugars, and excessive sodium, while increasing consumption of fruits, vegetables, whole grains, lean proteins, and healthy fats, individuals can help lower their risk of heart disease. A balanced meal plan can also contribute to maintaining healthy cholesterol levels and blood pressure.

5. Disease Prevention:

A comprehensive meal plan plays a crucial role in preventing various chronic diseases. By emphasizing nutrient-dense foods and limiting processed foods, individuals can reduce their risk of conditions such as obesity, type 2 diabetes, certain cancers, and hypertension. A balanced diet rich in fruits and vegetables provides antioxidants, which help protect against oxidative stress and cellular damage.

6. Improved Digestive Health:

A well-structured meal plan that includes ample fiber from whole grains, fruits, and vegetables can promote healthy digestion. Adequate fiber intake supports regular bowel movements, prevents constipation, and contributes to a healthy gut microbiome. This improves overall digestive health and may help reduce the risk of conditions such as diverticulitis and colorectal cancer.

7. Mental Well-being:

A comprehensive meal plan can positively impact mental health and cognitive functioning. Nutrient-dense foods provide essential nutrients and antioxidants that support brain function and improve mood. Balancing meals and snacks with complex carbohydrates, lean proteins, and healthy fats helps stabilize blood sugar levels, providing a consistent and steady supply of energy to the brain.

8. Convenience and Organization:

Following a comprehensive meal plan offers the benefit of convenience and organization. Planning meals in advance, including grocery shopping, meal prepping, and packing healthy snacks, saves time, reduces impulsive food choices, and ensures that nutritious options are readily available. This can help individuals maintain consistency in their eating habits and make healthier choices even during busy days.

Conclusion:

Adopting a comprehensive meal plan provides numerous benefits for overall health and well-being. From ensuring optimal nutrition and weight management to supporting blood sugar control, heart health, disease prevention, improved digestion, and mental well-being, a well-structured and balanced eating plan positively impacts various aspects of life. By working with a registered dietitian or nutritionist, individuals can develop a meal plan tailored to their specific needs, preferences, and goals, supporting long-term health and vitality.

Chapter 3. Building a Diabetes-Friendly Food List

Building a diabetes-friendly food list is a crucial step in managing blood sugar levels and preventing complications associated with diabetes. A well-rounded and balanced food list can provide individuals with diabetes the necessary tools to make informed and nutritious choices. This note will outline the key considerations for building a diabetes-friendly food list, including nutrient composition, portion control, glycemic index, and practical tips for creating a diverse and enjoyable meal plan.

1. Nutrient Composition:

a. **Carbohydrates**: Choose complex carbohydrates with a low glycemic index, which have a slower impact on blood sugar levels. Examples include whole grains (oats, quinoa, whole wheat), legumes (beans, lentils), and non-starchy vegetables (leafy greens, broccoli, peppers).

b. **Proteins**: Incorporate lean protein sources such as skinless poultry, fish, tofu, eggs, low-fat dairy products, and plant-based protein sources like beans, lentils, and nuts. Protein promotes satiety and blood sugar regulation.

c. **Healthy Fats:** Consume foods high in avocados, nuts, seeds, olive oil, and fatty fish like mackerel and salmon in moderation. They support heart health and offer vital nutrients.

d. Fiber: Focus on high-fiber foods like fruits, vegetables, whole grains, and legumes. Fiber slows down the digestion and absorption of carbohydrates, preventing blood sugar spikes and promoting digestive health.

2. Portion Control:

Understanding portion sizes is crucial for managing blood sugar levels effectively. Be mindful of portion control by using measuring tools or visual cues. For example:

a. Use a food scale to accurately measure servings.

b. Learn visual portion cues like a fist for carbohydrates, a palm for protein, and a thumb for fats.

c. Avoid super-sized portions and be mindful of calorie intake.

3. Glycemic Index and Load:

Consider the glycemic index (GI) and glycemic load (GL) of foods to help guide food choices and manage blood sugar levels.

a. Glycemic Index: The GI ranks carbohydrates based on how quickly they raise blood glucose levels. Choose foods with a low or moderate GI value (55 or less) to minimize blood sugar spikes.

b. Glycemic Load: The GL considers both the quality and quantity of carbohydrates in a serving. Foods with a low GL (10 or less) provide a gradual rise in blood sugar levels.

4. Practical Tips:

a. Create a Balanced Plate: Aim to make half of your plate non-starchy vegetables, one-quarter lean protein, and one-quarter whole grains or starchy vegetables.

b. Choose Whole Foods: Opt for whole, minimally processed foods whenever possible to maximize nutrition and minimize added sugars, sodium, and unhealthy fats.

c. Be Mindful of Added Sugars: Read food labels and avoid products with added sugars, high fructose corn syrup, and sweeteners. Look for alternative names for added sugars like dextrose, fructose, or maltose.

d. Stay Hydrated: Include water as the primary beverage and limit sugary drinks and juices.

e. Meal Planning: Plan meals and snacks ahead of time to ensure a balanced and varied intake throughout the day. This helps avoid impulsive and less healthy food choices.

f. Consult with a Registered Dietitian: Seek guidance from a registered dietitian specializing in diabetes to create a personalized food list that aligns with individual health goals and preferences.

Conclusion:

Building a diabetes-friendly food list is essential for managing blood sugar levels and promoting overall health. By incorporating nutrient-dense foods, practicing portion control, considering the glycemic index and load, and using practical tips, individuals with diabetes can create a diverse and enjoyable meal plan.Consulting with a registered dietitian specializing in diabetes can provide personalized guidance and support, ensuring the food list meets individual needs and preferences. Through mindful food choices and a well-structured eating plan, individuals can maintain stable blood sugar levels and reduce the risk of complications in diabetes.

Low-Glycemic Index Foods

Low-glycemic index flour refers to flour that has a lower impact on blood sugar levels compared to regular flour. It is particularly beneficial for individuals with diabetes or those looking to manage their blood sugar levels effectively. This comprehensive note will explore the concept of low-glycemic index flour, its advantages for blood sugar control, and popular options available in the market.

1. Understanding the Glycemic Index:
Carbohydrates are ranked on a glycemic index (GI) based on how quickly they raise blood glucose levels. Foods with a high GI (70 or above) are rapidly digested and absorbed, leading to a rapid increase in blood sugar levels. On the other hand, low GI foods (55 or below) are digested and

absorbed more gradually, resulting in a slower and more controlled blood sugar response.

2. Advantages of Low-Glycemic Index Flour:

Using low-glycemic index flour in baking or cooking offers several benefits, especially for individuals with diabetes or those seeking overall blood sugar control:

a.   Blood   Sugar   Management: Low-glycemic index flour helps stabilize blood sugar levels by providing a slower and more controlled release of glucose into the bloodstream. This prevents rapid fluctuations in blood sugar, reducing the risk of hyperglycemia and promoting better diabetes management.

b. Sustained Energy: Low-glycemic index flour provides sustained energy over a more extended period. It helps avoid the rapid rise and subsequent crash in blood sugar levels that can lead to feelings of fatigue and sluggishness.

c. Increased Satiety: Foods made with low-glycemic index flour tend to be more filling and satisfying. This can help control hunger and reduce the likelihood of overeating or snacking on high-glycemic index foods.

d. Weight Management: Due to its impact on stabilizing blood sugar levels and promoting satiety, low-glycemic index flour can be beneficial for weight management efforts. It can support appetite control, reduce cravings, and aid in weight loss or weight maintenance.

3. Examples of Low-Glycemic Index Flours:

Several types of flour have a lower glycemic index compared to traditional wheat flour. Examples include:

a. Whole Wheat Flour: Whole wheat flour is made from whole grains, including the bran, germ, and endosperm. It has a lower glycemic index than refined wheat flour since it retains the fiber content of the grain, which slows down the digestion and absorption of carbohydrates.

b. Almond Flour: Almond flour is a gluten-free, low-carbohydrate alternative made from finely ground almonds. It has a minimal impact on blood sugar levels and is rich in healthy fats, protein, and fiber.

c. Coconut Flour: Coconut flour is derived from dried coconut meat and is gluten-free. It has a low glycemic index, high fiber content, and adds a subtly sweet flavor to baked goods.

d. Chickpea Flour: Chickpea flour, also known as garbanzo bean flour, is made from ground chickpeas. It is gluten-free, rich in protein and fiber, and has a lower glycemic index compared to wheat flour.

e. Lentil Flour: Lentil flour is made from ground lentils and is packed with protein, fiber, and various essential nutrients. It has a low glycemic index and is a suitable option for baking or cooking.

4. Incorporating Low-Glycemic Index Flours:

When using low-glycemic index flour, it is essential to consider the following:

a. Recipe Modification: When substituting low-glycemic index flour for traditional wheat flour in recipes, adjustments may be necessary. These flours often have different textures, absorption rates, and binding properties.

b. Combination Approach: Mixing low-glycemic index flour with other flours or binders, such as whole wheat flour, oat flour, or flaxseed meal, can help achieve the desired texture and improve baking outcomes.

c. Portion Control: While low-glycemic index flours have a lower impact on blood sugar levels, portion control is still important. Monitoring serving sizes and overall carbohydrate intake is crucial for maintaining stable blood sugar levels.

d. Individual Preferences: Experimenting with different low-glycemic index flours can help individuals determine the flavors, textures, and baking properties that suit their taste preferences and dietary needs.

Conclusion:

Incorporating low-glycemic index flour into baking and cooking offers several advantages for blood sugar management, sustained energy, increased satiety, and weight management. Options such as whole wheat flour, almond flour, coconut flour, chickpea flour, and lentil flour provide alternative sources of nutrients and are beneficial for individuals with diabetes or those looking to maintain stable blood sugar levels. Careful consideration of recipes, portion control, and personal preferences helps ensure successful integration of low-glycemic index flour into a balanced and diabetes-friendly diet.

High-Fiber Foods

High-fiber foods play a crucial role in maintaining a healthy and balanced diet. Fiber is a type of carbohydrate that is not easily digested by the body, providing numerous health benefits. This comprehensive note will explore the importance of high-fiber foods, their various types, health benefits, and examples of foods rich in fiber.

1. Importance of High-Fiber Foods:

High-fiber foods are essential for overall health and well-being. Fiber offers numerous advantages, including:

a. Digestive Health: Fiber adds bulk to the diet, promoting regular bowel movements and preventing constipation. It can also aid in the prevention of digestive disorders such as diverticulitis and hemorrhoids.

b. Weight Management: High-fiber foods are often low in calories and provide a feeling of fullness and satiety, which can help manage weight by reducing overeating and controlling calorie intake.

c. Blood Sugar Control: Soluble fiber slows down the absorption of sugar, helping to regulate blood sugar levels. For people who already have diabetes or are at risk of getting it, this can be especially helpful.

d. Heart Health: Diets high in fiber, particularly soluble fiber, can help lower cholesterol by binding to and blocking the absorption of cholesterol in the digestive tract. Thus, the chance of developing heart disease is decreased.

e. Reduced Risk of Chronic Diseases: A high-fiber diet has been associated with a lower risk of developing chronic conditions such as obesity, type 2 diabetes, cardiovascular disease, and certain types of cancer, including colon and breast cancer.

2. Types of Fiber:
There are two types of dietary fiber:

a. Soluble Fiber: Soluble fiber dissolves in water, forming a gel-like substance in the digestive tract. It can help regulate blood sugar levels, lower cholesterol, and aid in weight management. Good sources of soluble fiber include oats, barley, legumes, fruits (e.g., apples, oranges, berries), and vegetables (e.g., carrots, Brussels sprouts).

b. Insoluble Fiber: Insoluble fiber does not dissolve in water and adds bulk to the diet. It helps with digestion, encourages regular bowel movements, and guards against constipation. Whole grains (such as wheat and brown rice), nuts, seeds, and the skins of fruits and vegetables are foods high in insoluble fiber.

3. Foods with a High Fiber Content:

It's critical to include a range of high-fiber foods in your diet. Here are a few foods high in fiber:

a. Whole Grains: Whole wheat bread, whole grain pasta, brown rice, quinoa, oats, and barley.

b. Legumes: Lentils, chickpeas, black beans, kidney beans, and split peas.

c. Fruits: Berries, apples, pears, oranges, bananas, and avocados.

d. Vegetables: Broccoli, Brussels sprouts, cauliflower, carrots, spinach, kale, and peas.

e. Nuts and Seeds: Almonds, walnuts, chia seeds, flaxseeds, and pumpkin seeds.

f. Bran: Wheat bran, oat bran, and rice bran.

4. Incorporating High-Fiber Foods:
To increase your fiber intake, follow these tips:

a. Gradual Increase: Increase fiber intake gradually to allow your body to adjust and minimize digestive discomfort.

b. Read Food Labels: Check the nutritional information on food labels to identify products that are high in fiber.

c. Choose Whole Foods: Opt for whole foods rather than processed foods, as they tend to contain more fiber and fewer added sugars.

d. Include a Variety: Aim to include a variety of high-fiber foods in your meals to obtain the full range of nutrients.

e. Hydration: Drink plenty of water throughout the day to help fiber move smoothly through the digestive tract.

5. Recommended Daily Fiber Intake:
The amount of fiber that should be consumed daily depends on factors like age, sex, and general health. Generally speaking, adults ought to strive for:

a. Men: 30-38 grams of fiber per day.

b. Women: 21-25 grams of fiber per day.
Conclusion:
Incorporating high-fiber foods into your diet is essential for promoting digestive health, maintaining a healthy weight,

controlling blood sugar levels, and reducing the risk of chronic diseases. Including a variety of fiber-rich foods, such as whole grains, legumes, fruits, vegetables, nuts, and seeds, can help you meet your daily fiber needs. Gradually increasing fiber intake, reading food labels, and opting for whole, unprocessed foods are key strategies for achieving a high-fiber diet. By prioritizing high-fiber foods, you can support your overall health and well-being.

Lean Proteins

Lean proteins are an essential component of a balanced diet, providing the body with vital nutrients and supporting various bodily functions. Incorporating lean proteins into meals offers numerous health benefits, including muscle growth and repair, weight management, satiety, and overall well-being. This comprehensive note will highlight the importance of lean proteins, their health benefits, and examples of lean protein sources.

1. Importance of Lean Proteins:
Lean proteins are an important part of a healthy diet for several reasons:

a. Muscle Growth and Repair: Protein is essential for building and repairing tissues, including muscles. Consuming an adequate amount of lean protein supports muscle growth and helps maintain muscle integrity.

b. Weight Management: Protein-rich foods are typically more satiating and can help control appetite, reducing the likelihood of overeating or snacking on unhealthy foods. A diet high in lean proteins can contribute to weight management and even weight loss.

c. Metabolism and Energy: Proteins are involved in numerous metabolic processes, including energy production. They provide a source of calories and can help stabilize blood sugar levels, preventing energy crashes.

d. Bone Health: Proteins play a role in maintaining bone health and preventing conditions like osteoporosis. Adequate protein intake, combined with other bone-building nutrients, supports bone density and overall skeletal strength.

e. Hormone and Enzyme Production: Proteins are the building blocks for various hormones and enzymes needed for the proper functioning of the body. These substances regulate important processes such as metabolism, digestion, and immune function.

2. Health Benefits of Lean Proteins:

Including lean proteins in your diet offers several health benefits:

a. Muscle Development and Maintenance: Adequate intake of lean proteins, in conjunction with regular exercise, promotes muscle growth, strength, and repair. This is crucial for maintaining a healthy body composition and functional mobility.

b. Satiety and Weight Management: Protein-rich foods tend to be more filling and can help control hunger and cravings. Including lean proteins in meals can aid in weight management by reducing calorie intake and promoting a sense of fullness.

c. Blood Sugar Control: Protein has a minimal impact on blood sugar levels compared to carbohydrates. Consuming lean proteins along with carbohydrates can slow down the absorption of sugar and regulate blood glucose levels, benefiting individuals with diabetes and supporting overall blood sugar control.

d. Heart Health: Lean proteins, such as fish, poultry without skin, legumes, and low-fat dairy products, are healthier alternatives to fatty meats and processed meats. They contribute to a heart-healthy diet by providing essential nutrients and minimizing saturated fat intake.

3. Examples of Lean Protein Sources:
Several foods are excellent sources of lean proteins:

a. Poultry: Skinless chicken breast, turkey breast, and lean cuts of turkey or chicken.

b. Fish: Salmon, trout, tuna, mackerel, and other fatty fish provide high-quality protein along with heart-healthy omega-3 fatty acids.

c. Legumes: Lentils, chickpeas, beans (black beans, kidney beans, navy beans), and edamame (soybeans) are plant-based sources of lean protein, as well as fiber.

d. Low-Fat Dairy: Greek yogurt, cottage cheese, and skim milk contain substantial amounts of protein without excessive fat content.

e. Eggs: Whole eggs or egg whites are a versatile and inexpensive source of lean protein.

f. Lean Meats: Lean cuts of beef, such as sirloin and tenderloin, or pork, such as tenderloin, can be included in moderation.

g. Tofu and Tempeh: These plant-based protein sources derived from soybeans can provide a protein-rich alternative for individuals following a vegetarian or vegan diet.

h. Nuts and Seeds: Almonds, walnuts, chia seeds, flaxseeds, and hemp seeds contribute to protein intake while also providing healthy fats and other nutrients.

4. Incorporating Lean Proteins:
To incorporate lean proteins into your diet:

a. Prioritize these protein sources in your meals and snacks.

b. Include a mix of animal and plant-based proteins for variety and additional health benefits.

c. Opt for cooking methods that minimize added fats, such as grilling, broiling, baking, or steaming.

d. Combine proteins with other nutrient-rich foods, such as vegetables, whole grains, and healthy fats, for a well-rounded meal.

e. If following a vegetarian or vegan diet, ensure you are combining complementary plant-based proteins to provide all essential amino acids.

5. Recommended Protein Intake:
The amount of protein that is advised varies based on age, sex, and degree of activity. As a general guideline, aim for:

a. Adults: 0.8 grams of protein per kilogram of body weight, or approximately 10-35% of daily caloric intake.

b. Athletes or those engaging in intense physical activity: 1.2-2.0 grams of protein per kilogram of body weight.

Conclusion:

Incorporating lean proteins into your diet is crucial for maintaining overall health and well-being. Lean proteins provide essential nutrients, support muscle growth, promote weight management, and offer numerous other health benefits. Including a variety of lean protein sources, such as poultry, fish, legumes, low-fat dairy, eggs, and plant-based proteins, provides a well-rounded and balanced diet. By making lean proteins a priority in your meals, you can support optimal health and enhance your overall nutritional intake. As always, individual protein needs may vary, so consult with a healthcare professional or registered dietitian to determine the appropriate protein intake for your specific needs.

Healthy Fats

It's not always true that fats are unhealthy for you. Good fats offer a host of health advantages and are a crucial component of a well-balanced diet. They are critical for preserving heart health, fostering brain function, supporting optimal body functions, and even helping with weight management. This extensive note will clarify the significance of healthy fats, their varieties, health advantages, and food examples that are high in healthy

1. Importance of Healthy Fats:
Healthy fats are crucial for our overall well-being due to the following reasons:

a. Energy Source: Fats are a concentrated source of energy, providing more than twice the energy density of carbohydrates or proteins. They serve as a vital fuel source, especially during periods of low carbohydrate intake or intense physical activity.

b. Nutrient Absorption: Some vitamins, such as vitamins A, D, E, and K, are fat-soluble, meaning they require fat for absorption. Consuming healthy fats helps ensure the adequate absorption of these essential vitamins.

c. Brain Function: The brain is composed mostly of fat, and healthy fats, particularly omega-3 fatty acids, are crucial for brain development, function, and cognitive health. They may contribute to improved memory, focus, and mental well-being.

d. Heart Health: Certain types of healthy fats, such as monounsaturated and polyunsaturated fats, can help improve cholesterol levels, reduce inflammation, and lower the risk of heart disease and stroke.

e. Hormone Regulation: Fats play a role in hormone production and regulation. Maintaining a balanced intake of healthy fats can support hormonal balance and overall reproductive health.

2. Types of Healthy Fats:
There are different types of healthy fats, each offering unique health benefits. These include:

a. Monounsaturated Fats: Found in foods such as olive oil, avocados, nuts (almonds, cashews, peanuts), and seeds (sesame seeds, pumpkin seeds). Monounsaturated fats can help reduce bad cholesterol levels and lower the risk of heart disease.

b. Polyunsaturated Fats: These fats include omega-3 and omega-6 fatty acids. Walnuts, flaxseeds, chia seeds, and fatty fish (salmon, mackerel, and sardines) are good sources of omega-3 fatty acids. Omega-6 fatty acids are found in vegetable oils (corn, soybean, sunflower) and nuts. Both types of fatty acids are essential for brain health, reducing inflammation, and supporting heart health.

c. Omega-3 Fatty Acids: In addition to fatty fish, omega-3 fatty acids can also be obtained from algae-based supplements, krill oil, and fortified foods. They have been associated with a reduced risk of heart disease, improved brain function, and reduced inflammation.

d. Saturated Fats (in Moderation): While saturated fats should be consumed in moderation, not all saturated fats are considered harmful. Some foods that contain saturated fats, such as coconut oil and dark chocolate, also provide additional health benefits. Coconut oil is rich in medium-chain triglycerides (MCTs), which are metabolized differently and can have positive effects on weight management and cognitive function.

3. Health Benefits of Healthy Fats:
Consuming healthy fats as part of a balanced diet offers several health benefits, including:

a.   Heart   Health: Including monounsaturated and polyunsaturated fats in the diet has been associated with a lower risk of heart disease and improved lipid profiles. These fats have the ability to raise HDL cholesterol levels and decrease LDL cholesterol, the bad kind of cholesterol.

b. Brain Health: Omega-3 fatty acids, particularly docosahexaenoic acid (DHA), are essential for optimal brain development, function, and mental well-being. Adequate intake of omega-3 fatty acids has been linked to a reduced risk of cognitive decline and age-related disorders such as Alzheimer's disease.

c. Weight Management: Healthy fats contribute to satiety and can help control cravings, reducing the likelihood of overeating. They also aid in the absorption of fat-soluble vitamins, which play a role in weight management and overall health.

d. Inflammation Reduction: Omega-3 fatty acids and other healthy fats have anti-inflammatory properties, which can help reduce chronic inflammation in the body. Chronic inflammation is associated with various diseases, including heart disease and certain types of cancer.

4. Examples of Foods with Healthy Fats: Incorporate the following foods into your diet to ensure an adequate intake of healthy fats:

a. Avocados: Avocados are rich in monounsaturated fats, fiber, and various vitamins and minerals.

b. Fatty Fish: Salmon, mackerel, sardines, and trout are excellent sources of omega-3 fatty acids, which support heart health and brain function.

c. Nuts and Seeds: Almonds, walnuts, chia seeds, flaxseeds, and pumpkin seeds provide a combination of healthy fats, fiber, and other essential nutrients.

d. Olive Oil: Extra virgin olive oil is an excellent source of monounsaturated fats and antioxidants, known to support heart health and reduce inflammation.

e. Coconut Oil: Although high in saturated fats, coconut oil contains beneficial medium-chain triglycerides (MCTs) that can provide energy and support weight management.

f. Dark Chocolate: Dark chocolate with a high cocoa content contains healthy fats, antioxidants, and minerals, providing potential cardiovascular benefits.

5. Incorporating Healthy Fats:
To incorporate healthy fats into your diet:

a. Choose Olive Oil: Swap out less healthy cooking oils for extra virgin olive oil when preparing meals.

b. Add Avocado: Include avocado in salads, sandwiches, or as a spread alternative to butter or mayonnaise.

c. Eat Fatty Fish: Aim to consume fatty fish at least twice a week to obtain a good supply of omega-3 fatty acids.

d. Snack on Nuts and Seeds: Incorporate nuts and seeds as snacks or sprinkle them onto salads, yogurt, or oatmeal.

e. Moderate Coconut Oil: Use coconut oil occasionally in cooking or baking, but be mindful of its high saturated fat content.

f. Enjoy Dark Chocolate: Opt for dark chocolate with a high percentage of cocoa (70% or more) as an occasional treat.

Conclusion:

Incorporating healthy fats into your diet is crucial for maintaining optimal health and well-being. Healthy fats provide essential nutrients, support heart health, promote brain function, and even aid in weight management. Including a variety of healthy fats from sources such as avocados, fatty fish, nuts, seeds, olive oil, and dark chocolate can enhance the nutritional value of your meals. As always, it is important to consume healthy fats in moderation as part of a well-balanced diet. Consult a healthcare professional or registered dietitian for personalized advice on incorporating healthy fats into your diet and to determine the appropriate intake for your specific needs.

Non-Starchy Vegetables

Non-starchy vegetables play a crucial role in a healthy and balanced diet. These vegetables are low in calories and carbohydrates while being packed with essential nutrients, fiber, and antioxidants. Including non-starchy vegetables in meals offers numerous health benefits, such as weight management, improved digestion, lowered risk of chronic diseases, and overall vitality. This comprehensive note will highlight the importance of non-starchy vegetables, their health benefits, and provide examples of non-starchy vegetables.

1. Importance of Non-Starchy Vegetables: Non-starchy vegetables are an important component of a nutritious diet for several reasons:

a.   Nutrient Density: Non-starchy vegetables are rich in vitamins, minerals, and phytochemicals, making them excellent sources of essential nutrients. They contribute to overall health and provide valuable antioxidants that help protect the body against oxidative stress and inflammation.

b. Fiber Content: Non-starchy vegetables are an excellent source of dietary fiber, which aids in digestion, supports regular bowel movements, and helps maintain gut health. Fiber also contributes to a feeling of fullness, making non-starchy vegetables beneficial for weight management and appetite control.

c. Low Calorie and Carbohydrate Content: Non-starchy vegetables are naturally low in calories and carbohydrates, making them an ideal food choice for those looking to manage their weight or control their blood sugar levels. They provide important nutrients without significantly impacting caloric intake or blood glucose levels.

d. Hydration: Many non-starchy vegetables, such as cucumbers and leafy greens, have high water content, contributing to hydration and promoting healthy skin and overall cellular function.

e. Disease Prevention: Non-starchy vegetables have been associated with a reduced risk of chronic diseases, including heart disease, certain types of cancer, and obesity. The antioxidant and anti-inflammatory compounds found in non-starchy vegetables may help protect against these diseases.

2. Health Benefits of Non-Starchy Vegetables:

Including non-starchy vegetables in your diet offers several health benefits:

a. Weight Management: Non-starchy vegetables provide bulk and fiber without adding excessive calories. They help create a feeling of fullness and satiation, reducing the likelihood of overeating and aiding in weight management.

b. Digestive Health: The fiber content in non-starchy vegetables supports a healthy digestive system by preventing constipation, promoting regular bowel movements, and nourishing beneficial gut bacteria. This may help with better nutrient absorption and digestion.

c. Heart Health: Non-starchy vegetables have been associated with a reduced risk of heart disease due to their fiber and nutrient content. The antioxidants found in these vegetables can also help lower blood pressure and inflammation, promoting cardiovascular health.

d. Blood Sugar Control: Non-starchy vegetables have a minimal impact on blood sugar levels due to their low carbohydrate content. Including non-starchy vegetables in meals can help stabilize blood sugar levels and manage conditions such as diabetes.

e. Protection against Chronic Diseases: The antioxidants and phytochemicals present in non-starchy vegetables have been shown to have anti-cancer properties, reduce the risk of certain types of cancer, and protect against other chronic diseases, such as age-related macular degeneration.

3. Examples of Non-Starchy Vegetables:

Here are examples of non-starchy vegetables that can be incorporated into a balanced diet:

a. **Leafy Greens**: Spinach, kale, lettuce, Swiss chard, and arugula are nutrient-dense and provide a variety of vitamins, minerals, and antioxidants.

b. **Cruciferous Vegetables**: Broccoli, cauliflower, Brussels sprouts, cabbage, and bok choy are rich in vitamins, fiber, and cancer-fighting compounds.

c. **Bell Peppers**: Red, green, and yellow bell peppers offer a good source of vitamins A and C, as well as antioxidants.

d. Cucumbers: Cucumbers have a high water content, making them refreshing and hydrating. They are also low in calories and provide fiber.

e. Tomatoes: Tomatoes are rich in lycopene, an antioxidant that may reduce the risk of certain cancers. They supply vitamins A and C as well.

f. Zucchini: A wonderful complement to many meals, zucchini is low in calories and carbs. It's a healthy supply of vitamin C and fiber.

g. Asparagus: Packed with fiber, folate, vitamins A, C, E, and K, and other nutrients, asparagus is a super food. It functions as a natural diuretic as well.

h. Mushrooms: Mushrooms are low in calories and carbohydrates while providing important nutrients, including potassium and B vitamins.

4.   Incorporating   Non-Starchy Vegetables:

To incorporate non-starchy vegetables into your diet:

a. Fill Half Your Plate: Aim to fill at least half of your plate with non-starchy vegetables during meals.

b. Variety is Key: Include a variety of non-starchy vegetables to ensure you obtain a wide range of nutrients and antioxidants.

c. Raw or Cooked: Non-starchy vegetables can be enjoyed raw in salads, as snacks, or lightly cooked through methods such as steaming, sautéing, roasting, or grilling.

d. Add to Recipes: Incorporate non-starchy vegetables into recipes such as stir-fries, soups, omelets, casseroles, or pasta dishes to increase their nutritional value and add color and flavor.

e. Try Smoothies and Juices: Add non-starchy vegetables like spinach or kale to smoothies or juices for an added nutritional boost.

5. Recommended Daily Intake:

There's no specific recommended daily intake for non-starchy vegetables, but the general guideline is to consume 2-3 cups (4-6 servings) of non-starchy vegetables per day. Adjustments may be needed based on individual needs and dietary goals.

Conclusion:

Non-starchy vegetables are a vital component of a healthy diet, providing essential nutrients, fiber, and antioxidants. Incorporating a variety of non-starchy vegetables into meals supports weight management, promotes optimal digestion, reduces the risk of chronic diseases, and contributes to overall vitality. Including leafy greens, cruciferous vegetables, bell peppers, cucumbers, tomatoes, zucchini, asparagus, mushrooms, and other non-starchy vegetables can enhance the nutritional value and taste of your meals. Strive to include non-starchy vegetables in your daily diet for optimal health and wellness.

Foods to Limit or Avoid

Managing diabetes requires maintaining a balanced and nutritious diet. It is essential to be mindful of the foods you consume as certain foods can significantly impact blood sugar levels. In this comprehensive note, we will discuss the foods that are best limited or avoided for individuals with diabetes.

1. **Sugary Foods and Beverages:** Foods high in added sugars and refined carbohydrates should be limited. These include soda, fruit juices, energy drinks, sweets, pastries, and desserts. Consuming these foods can cause rapid spikes in blood sugar levels, making it difficult to manage diabetes effectively.

2. **Processed Carbohydrates:** Refined grains and processed carbohydrates such as white bread, pasta, and rice often lack fiber and contain added sugars. These foods are quickly digested and can lead to sharp increases in blood sugar levels. Opt for whole grains like quinoa, brown rice, and whole-wheat bread, as they are higher in fiber and have a slower impact on blood sugar.

3. **Sweetened Yogurts and Fruit Juices:** Many yogurts and fruit juices are marketed as healthy options, but they

often contain added sugars. Check labels and choose unsweetened or plain versions instead. Additionally, it's better to consume whole fruits rather than fruit juices, as they contain more fiber and can have a lower impact on blood sugar levels.

4. High-Fat Animal Products: While lean meats like skinless chicken and turkey can be part of a healthy diabetes diet, it's important to moderate the consumption of high-fat animal products. Red meat, processed meats (such as sausages and bacon), and full-fat dairy products can contribute to increased cardiovascular risks. Opt for lean cuts of meat and choose low-fat dairy products or plant-based alternatives.

5. Trans Fats and Saturated Fats: Foods high in trans fats and saturated fats can lead to elevated cholesterol levels and increase the risk of heart disease. Avoid fried foods, commercially baked goods, and processed snacks like chips, cookies, and pastries that may contain trans fats. Limit the intake of saturated fats by choosing lean proteins, low-fat dairy products, and healthier fats found in sources like avocados, nuts, seeds, and olive oil.

6. **Sugar-Sweetened Beverages**: Regular consumption of sugary beverages is strongly associated with obesity and an increased risk of developing type 2 diabetes. These include soda, sweetened tea, sports drinks, and other sugary drinks. Opt for water, unsweetened tea or coffee, or naturally flavored water with no added sugars.

7. **Alcohol**: While moderate alcohol consumption is typically considered safe for some individuals with diabetes, excessive intake can lead to unstable

blood sugar levels and hinder diabetes management. It is important to monitor your blood sugar levels when consuming alcoholic beverages and keep within the recommended guidelines for moderate consumption.

Remember, a well-balanced and varied diet is key for managing diabetes effectively. It is always advisable to consult a registered dietitian or healthcare professional to tailor a personalized meal plan based on individual needs and preferences.

Take control of your diabetes through mindful food choices, regular physical activity, and regular check-ups with your healthcare provider. Living a healthy lifestyle can make a significant impact on diabetes management and overall well-being.

Chapter 4. Creating a Comprehensive Diabetes Meal Plan

As an AI language model, I can provide you with a comprehensive diabetes meal plan. However, it's important to note that I'm not a certified nutritionist or a healthcare professional. It would be best to consult with a registered dietitian or healthcare provider to tailor a meal plan specifically for your needs.

Here is a sample meal plan to help you manage diabetes:

Breakfast:
- **Option 1:** 1 cup of cooked oatmeal topped with berries and a tablespoon of almond butter.

- **Option 2**: Veggie omelet made with egg whites, spinach, bell peppers, and tomatoes, along with a side of whole wheat toast.

- **Option 3**: Greek yogurt with sliced almonds and a small portion of mixed fruits.

Mid-morning Snack:

- **Option 1**: A small apple with a tablespoon of peanut butter.

Option 2: A small handful of mixed seeds and nuts.

- **Third option**: Hummus on carrot sticks.

Lunch options include grilled chicken breast, steamed vegetables, and quinoa on the side.

- **Option 2:** Salad with mixed greens, grilled salmon, cherry tomatoes, cucumber slices, and a low-fat vinaigrette dressing.

- **Option 3**: Turkey wrap with whole wheat tortilla, lettuce, tomato, avocado, and mustard.

Afternoon Snack:
- **Option 1**: Celery sticks with a tablespoon of almond butter.
- **Option 2**: Cucumber slices with a small portion of low-fat cottage cheese.
- **Option 3**: Hard-boiled eggs and a handful of cherry tomatoes.

Dinner:
- **Option 1**: Steamed broccoli, roasted sweet potatoes, and baked salmon.
- **Option 2**: Grilled lean steak with quinoa and asparagus.
- **Option 3**: Stir-fried tofu with mixed vegetables and brown rice.

Evening Snack:

- **Option 1**: Sugar-free yogurt with a sprinkle of cinnamon.

- **Option 2**: Air-popped popcorn.

- **Option 3**: Sliced bell peppers with hummus.

It's important to note that portion sizes and individual nutritional requirements may vary. Make sure to monitor your blood glucose levels, and adapt the meal plan as needed. Always remember that for individualized advice, it's best to speak with a healthcare professional.

Balancing Macronutrients: Carbohydrates, Proteins, and Fats

Maintaining a healthy diet involves balancing your intake of macronutrients (carbohydrates, proteins, and fats) as well as incorporating essential micronutrients (vitamins and minerals) into your meals. Properly balancing these components is crucial for overall health, energy levels, and disease prevention. Here are some guidelines to help you achieve a well-rounded and balanced diet.

1. Micronutrients:
Micronutrients are essential for a number of biological processes. To ensure you get

an adequate supply of these nutrients, follow these tips:

- Include a variety of fruits and vegetables in your meals to obtain a wide range of vitamins and minerals.

- Opt for colorful options such as leafy greens, berries, citrus fruits, and sweet potatoes, as they are rich in antioxidants and phytochemicals.

- Don't overcook vegetables, as it can lead to nutrient loss. Aim for steaming or lightly sautéing them to preserve their nutritional value.

- Consider including whole grains, lean meats, dairy products, and legumes as they contain essential vitamins and minerals.

2. Carbohydrates:

An essential source of energy for the body is glucose. Here's how to balance your carbohydrate intake:

- Choose complex carbohydrates over simple carbohydrates. Whole grains, legumes, and vegetables provide a sustained release of energy and are rich in fiber, vitamins, and minerals.

- Limit consumption of refined carbohydrates like white bread, sugary drinks, pastries, and processed foods, as they can lead to blood sugar spikes and weight gain.

- Portion control is crucial. Aim to fill a quarter of your plate with carbohydrates during meals.

3. Proteins:

Proteins are essential for tissue repair, hormone production, and maintaining muscle mass. Follow these guidelines to balance your protein intake:

- Incorporate low-fat dairy products, fish, poultry, eggs, tofu, and legumes as sources of lean protein.
- Distribute protein intake throughout the day to aid in muscle repair and synthesis.
- For optimal nutrient intake, combine proteins with whole grains or vegetables to create balanced and complete meals.

4. Fats:

Dietary fats are necessary for healthy cell function, hormone production, and nutrient absorption.
- Focus on consuming healthy fats, such as avocados, nuts, seeds, olive oil, and fatty fish, which provide omega-3 fatty acids that support heart health.
- Limit saturated fats found in red meat, high-fat dairy products, and fried foods,

as they can raise cholesterol levels and increase the risk of heart disease.

- Balance your fat intake by opting for moderate portion sizes and choosing a combination of healthy fats.

Conclusion:

Achieving a balance of micronutrients, carbohydrates, proteins, and fats is crucial for maintaining a healthy diet. Prioritize incorporating a variety of colorful fruits and vegetables, whole grains, lean proteins, and healthy fats into your meals. Remember, portion control, diversity, and moderation are key. If you have specific dietary needs or health concerns, it's advisable to consult a registered dietitian for personalized guidance.

Portion Control and Meal Timing

Portion control and meal timing are key factors to consider for maintaining a healthy diet and managing weight. Properly controlling portion sizes and timing meals throughout the day can help promote satiety, prevent overeating, and optimize nutrient absorption. Here's a comprehensive guide to mastering portion control and meal timing for a healthy lifestyle.

1. Understanding Portion Control:

- Familiarize yourself with proper portion sizes by referring to visual cues, such as using your hand or everyday objects as a reference. For example:

  - A serving of meat should be roughly the size of your palm.

- A serving of grains or starchy foods (rice, pasta, etc.) should fit in your cupped hand.

- A serving of fats or oils should be equivalent to the size of your thumb.

- Read nutrition labels to determine appropriate portion sizes and adjust your servings accordingly.

- To aid with portion control visually, use smaller bowls and plates. By creating the appearance of a larger plate, this encourages eating less food. Eat mindfully by slowing down, enjoying every bite, and being aware of your body's signals of hunger and fullness. This aids in avoiding overindulging.

2. Timing Your Meals: To ensure that your body can adequately digest and absorb nutrients, try to eat three balanced meals a day at regular intervals. Refrain from missing meals, particularly breakfast, as it powers your metabolism and gives you energy for the day.

- Hacken to your body when you feel hungry and listen to fullness sign but be mindful of portion size when eating.

- Avoid late-night snacking, as it can disrupt sleep and lead to weight gain. If you're genuinely hungry, opt for a small, nutritious snack rather than high-calorie, processed foods.

3. Balancing Macronutrients:

- Include a balance of carbohydrates, proteins, and fats in each meal to provide energy and promote satiety.

- Opt for complex carbohydrates like whole grains, fruits, and vegetables, as they provide sustained energy and fiber.

- Ensure an adequate protein intake by incorporating lean sources such as poultry, fish, legumes, and tofu. - Select healthy fats from foods such as olive oil, avocados, nuts, and seeds. They promote general health and help with satiety.

4. **Hydration**: To stay hydrated, sip water throughout the day.

. It's best to sip water between meals rather than with meals to avoid diluting stomach acids and hindering the digestion process.

Conclusion:

Mastering portion control and meal timing is vital for maintaining a healthy diet. By understanding portion sizes, practicing mindful eating, and following a consistent meal timing routine, you can optimize your nutrient intake, manage weight, and promote overall well-being. Remember, each person's needs may vary, so it's always beneficial to consult with a registered dietitian for personalized guidance and recommendations

Incorporating Regular Physical Activity

I am writing to provide you with a comprehensive note on how incorporating regular physical activity can help you manage diabetes. Physical activity plays a crucial role in diabetes management and can have a significant positive impact on your overall health and well-being.

1. Understanding Diabetes:

Diabetes is a chronic condition characterized by high blood glucose levels due to either insufficient insulin production or improper utilization of insulin by the body. Regular physical activity can help manage diabetes by improving insulin sensitivity, controlling blood glucose levels, maintaining a healthy weight, reducing the risk of cardiovascular complications, and enhancing overall physical and mental health.

2. Benefits of Regular Physical Activity for Diabetes Management:

a. Improved Insulin Sensitivity: Physical activity helps your body use insulin more efficiently, leading to better blood sugar control. It enables your cells to take up glucose from the bloodstream and utilize it for energy.

b. Blood Sugar Control: Regular exercise can lower blood glucose levels by stimulating glucose uptake and utilization by the muscles. This may lessen the likelihood of abrupt increases or decreases in blood sugar.

c. Weight Management: Physical activity helps with weight loss or weight maintenance, which is crucial for managing diabetes. Being overweight increases the risk of developing insulin resistance and complicates blood sugar regulation.

d. **Cardiovascular Health**: Diabetes increases the risk of heart disease. Regular exercise helps improve cardiovascular health by reducing blood pressure, improving blood lipid profile, and strengthening the heart.

e. **Stress Reduction**: Exercise is a natural stress reliever, and managing stress is essential for diabetes management. Regular physical activity can help reduce stress levels, improve mood, and enhance overall mental well-being.

f. **Reduced Risk of Complications**: Engaging in regular physical activity can reduce the risk of complications associated with diabetes, such as neuropathy, kidney disease, and diabetic retinopathy.

3. Types of Physical Activity:

a. Aerobic Exercises: These activities increase your heart rate and breathing. Walking quickly, running, biking, swimming, and dancing are a few examples. Try to get in at least 150 minutes a week of aerobic activity at a moderate level.

b. Strength training: This type of exercise increases insulin resistance while also helping to build muscle. Bodyweight exercises, resistance bands, and weightlifting are a few examples.

Perform strength training exercises at least two days a week, targeting major muscle groups.

c. Flexibility Exercises: Stretching exercises improve flexibility, balance, and joint mobility. Incorporate stretching exercises at least two to three days a week.

d. Balance Exercises: These activities help prevent falls and improve stability. Examples include Tai Chi or yoga.

4. Getting Started:

a. Consult with Your Healthcare Team: Before starting any exercise routine, consult your healthcare team to receive personalized recommendations and ensure that your exercise plan aligns with your health status and any existing complications.

b. Start Slowly and Gradually Increase Intensity: If you are new to exercise, start with low-impact activities and gradually increase the duration and intensity over time. This approach will help prevent injuries and allow your body to adjust.

c. Monitor Blood Glucose Levels: Regularly monitor your blood glucose levels before, during, and after exercise. This will help you understand how your body responds and allow you to make appropriate adjustments to your diabetes management plan.

d. Stay Hydrated: To avoid dehydration, sip lots of water prior to, during, and after physical activity.. Avoid consuming sugary beverages that can cause blood sugar spikes.

e. Wear Appropriate Footwear: Choose well-fitting, comfortable athletic shoes to protect your feet and reduce the risk of foot ulcers or injuries.

Remember, regular physical activity should be part of an overall diabetes management plan that includes a healthy diet, medication (if prescribed), regular monitoring of blood glucose levels, and regular check-ups with your healthcare team.

In conclusion, incorporating regular physical activity into your routine is a key component of managing diabetes effectively. It offers numerous benefits, including improved insulin sensitivity, better blood sugar control, weight management, cardiovascular health, stress reduction, and reduced risk of complications. Start slowly, consult your healthcare team, and gradually increase the intensity and duration of your exercise routine. Stay motivated, listen to your body, and monitor your blood glucose levels to ensure safe and effective diabetes management.

Sample Diabetes Meal Plan

I understand that you are looking for a comprehensive sample meal plan for individuals with diabetes. It's essential to customize meal plans based on personal preferences, dietary restrictions, medication requirements, and health goals. However, here is an example of a balanced diabetes meal plan that can help maintain stable blood sugar levels and promote overall well-being.

Please note that it's always advisable to consult with a registered dietitian or healthcare provider for a personalized meal plan.

Meal Plan:

Breakfast:

- 1 boiled egg
- 1 slice whole-grain toast with sugar-free peanut butter
- 1 small apple
- 1 cup unsweetened Greek yogurt
- Coffee or tea without sugar

Mid-Morning Snack:

- A handful of unsalted nuts (almonds, walnuts, or pistachios)

- 1 small carrot or cucumber, sliced

Lunch:

- Grilled chicken breast (3 oz)

- One cup of brown rice or cooked quinoa

- Grilled vegetables such as broccoli, zucchini, and bell peppers

- 1 side salad with spinach, tomatoes, and a tablespoon of olive oil and vinegar dressing

- Unsweetened iced tea or water

Afternoon Snack:

- Sticks of celery dipped in nut butter or hummus

- 1 small orange

Dinner:

- Baked salmon (3 oz)

- 1/2 cup cooked whole wheat pasta with tomato sauce

- Steamed asparagus or green beans

- Mixed green salad with cucumbers, tomatoes, and vinaigrette dressing

- Water or herbal tea (unsweetened)

Evening Snack:

- Sugar-free yogurt with a sprinkle of nuts or berries

- Herbal tea

Bedtime Snack (if needed):

- 1 small handful of unsalted almonds or cashews

- Water

Please note that portion sizes and specific foods may need to be adjusted based on individual needs, preferences, and health goals. It's crucial to prioritize whole, unprocessed foods, limit added sugars, and focus on high-fiber sources.

General Tips:

1. Stay hydrated by drinking a lot of water all day.

2. Opt for low or non-fat dairy products.

3. Include a variety of colorful vegetables and fruits.

4. Choose complex carbohydrates such as whole grains, legumes, and starchy vegetables.

5. Consume lean sources of protein like poultry, fish, tofu, or legumes.

6. Limit or avoid sugary beverages, processed foods, and foods high in saturated and trans fats.

Remember, it is essential to monitor blood glucose levels regularly and adjust the meal plan accordingly. Work closely with a healthcare professional or a registered dietitian to develop a personalized diabetes meal plan that suits your individual needs.

Chapter 5. Breakfast Ideas for Diabetes

I understand that you are seeking breakfast ideas specifically catered to individuals with diabetes. Designing a balanced breakfast is crucial for managing blood sugar levels and providing sustained energy throughout the day. Below, I have compiled a list of healthy and delicious breakfast options that align with diabetes-friendly dietary guidelines.

1. Greek Yogurt Parfait:

- 1 cup nonfat Greek yogurt (unsweetened)

- 1/4 cup of fresh raspberries, strawberries, and blueberries

- One tablespoon of finely chopped nuts (pistachios, walnuts, or almonds)

- A sprinkle of cinnamon (optional)

2. Oatmeal with Fresh Fruit:

- 1/2 cup rolled oats (unflavored)

- 1 cup unsweetened almond milk or water

- 1/2 cup mixed fresh berries or sliced banana

- 1 tablespoon chopped nuts or seeds (such as chia or flaxseed)

- A drizzle of honey or a sprinkle of cinnamon (optional)

3. Vegetable Omelet:

- 2 egg whites and 1 whole egg, whisked

- 1/4 cup chopped vegetables (spinach, bell peppers, onions, or mushrooms)

- 1 ounce reduced-fat cheese (cheddar or feta)

- 1 slice whole-grain toast (optional)

4. Avocado Toast:

- 1 slice whole-grain bread, toasted

- 1/4 avocado, mashed

- Sliced tomatoes

- A generous squeeze of lemon juice

- A sprinkle of black pepper and sea salt

5. Cottage Cheese with Fruit:

- 1/2 cup low-fat cottage cheese

- 1/2 cup mixed fresh fruit (such as pineapple, melon, or grapes)

- 1 tablespoon of optionally chopped nuts or seeds

6. Smoothie Bowl:

- 1/2 cup unsweetened almond milk or low-fat yogurt

- 1/2 cup frozen berries (blueberries, strawberries, or raspberries)

- 1/4 banana

- 1 tablespoon nut butter (almond or peanut butter)
- A small handful of kale or spinach
- One tablespoon of flax or chia seeds
- Toppings: sliced fruits, nuts, seeds, or shredded coconut

Please remember to customize these options based on personal preferences, dietary restrictions, and carbohydrate counting if required. It's also beneficial to consult a registered dietitian or healthcare professional for an individualized meal plan.

General tips for a diabetes-friendly breakfast:

1. Include a source of lean protein (such as eggs, Greek yogurt, or cottage cheese) to promote satiety.

2. Incorporate high-fiber foods (oats, whole-grain bread, fruits, and vegetables) to help regulate blood sugar levels.

3. Stay hydrated by drinking water, unsweetened tea, or coffee.

4. Limit or avoid sugary beverages, processed breakfast cereals, and high-sugar spreads or jams.

Remember, managing diabetes involves a holistic approach, including regular physical activity and medications as prescribed. If you have any further questions or need additional guidance, consult a doctor.

Balanced and Nutrient-Dense Options

Maintaining a balanced and nutrient-dense diet is crucial for overall health and well-being. The body receives the vital nutrients, vitamins, and minerals it needs from a balanced diet to function at its best. It is essential to understand the concept of a balance between different food groups and incorporate nutrient-dense options into our meals. In this note, we will explore the importance of balance and nutrient-dense options and provide some practical tips to achieve them.

I. What is a Balanced Diet?

A balanced diet refers to the consumption of a variety of foods in appropriate proportions to meet the body's nutritional needs. It involves including foods from all major food groups, including fruits, vegetables, grains, protein sources, and dairy products. Each food group offers unique nutrients necessary for good health.

II. Understanding Nutrient-Dense Foods:
Nutrient-dense foods are those that provide a high concentration of essential nutrients relative to their calorie content. These foods are rich in vitamins, minerals, fiber, and phytochemicals while being relatively low in added sugars, unhealthy fats, and sodium. Nutrient-dense options should form the basis of a healthy diet.

III. Importance of Balance and Nutrient-Dense Options:

1. Optimal Nutrient Intake: A balanced and nutrient-dense diet ensures the intake of all essential nutrients, including macronutrients (carbohydrates, proteins, and fats) and micronutrients (vitamins and minerals). This supports a healthy immune system, proper growth, and development, and reduces the risk of chronic diseases.

2. Weight Management: Incorporating nutrient-dense options into a balanced diet helps manage weight effectively. These foods tend to be lower in calories while providing satiety, reducing the likelihood of overeating.

3. Boosts Energy Levels: Nutrient-dense foods provide sustained energy and prevent energy crashes due to their optimal combination of macronutrients, vitamins, and minerals.

4. Supports Overall Health: A balanced diet with nutrient-dense options plays a vital role in reducing the risk of various health conditions, including heart disease, obesity, diabetes, and certain cancers.

IV. Tips for Achieving Balance and Nutrient-Dense Options:

1. **Focus on Whole Foods**: Incorporate a variety of whole foods, such as fruits, vegetables, whole grains, lean proteins, and low-fat dairy, as they tend to be more nutrient-dense compared to processed foods.

2. **Portion Control**: Practice portion control to ensure balanced meals. Arrange a half portion of your plate with fruits and vegetables, a quarter with lean protein, and a quarter with starchy vegetables or whole grains.

3. **Read Food Labels**: Check food labels for hidden sugars, unhealthy fats, and excessive sodium content. Choose foods with shorter ingredient lists and recognizable ingredients.

4. **Limit Added Sugars and Unhealthy Fats**: Minimize the intake of sugary beverages, processed snacks, and deep-fried foods, as they tend to be low in

nutrients and high in added sugars and unhealthy fats.

5. Prioritize Variety: Experiment with different foods from each food group to ensure a wide variety of nutrients in your diet.

Conclusion:

Creating a balance with nutrient-dense options is essential for maintaining optimal health. Prioritizing whole foods, portion control, and making mindful choices can help achieve this balance. By incorporating a variety of nutrient-dense foods into our diet, we can fuel our bodies with essential nutrients, boost our overall well-being, and reduce the risk of chronic diseases.

Quick and Easy Breakfast Recipes

It's common to hear that breakfast is the most significant meal of the day. However, many people find themselves rushing through their mornings and compromising on the quality of their breakfast. To make things easier, we have compiled a list of quick and easy breakfast recipes that are both delicious and nutritious. These recipes require minimal time and effort, ensuring you can start your day off right without any hassle.

1. Overnight Chia Pudding:
Ingredients:
- 2 tablespoons chia seeds
- 1 cup milk (dairy or plant-based)
- 1 tablespoon honey or maple syrup

- Granola, almonds, or fresh fruit as a topping

Instructions:

1. In a jar or a bowl, combine the chia seeds, milk, and sweetener.

2. Stir well to prevent any clumps.

3. Place the mixture in the refrigerator overnight or for at least 3-4 hours.

4. Before serving, give the pudding a good stir and top it with your favorite fruits, nuts, or granola.

Benefits: Chia seeds are rich in fiber, Omega-3 fatty acids, and antioxidants, making this a healthy and filling breakfast option.

2. Avocado Toast:

Ingredients:

- 1 ripe avocado

- 2 slices of whole-grain bread

- Salt and pepper to taste

- Optional toppings: cherry tomatoes, feta cheese, poached egg, or smoked salmon

Instructions:

1. Toast the bread until golden and crispy.

2. Halve and pit the avocado, then scoop out the flesh into a bowl.

3. Use a fork to mash the avocado until it's smooth.

4. Evenly distribute the mashed avocado over the toast.

5. Add any desired toppings and season with salt and pepper.

Benefits: Avocados are a nutrient-dense way to start the day because they are full of vitamins, minerals, and healthy fats. Fiber and long-lasting energy are provided by the whole-grain bread.

3. Yogurt Confection:

Components:

- One cup of plain or flavored Greek yogurt

- 1/4 cup of nuts or granola - Sliced fruit or fresh berries

- Optional: honey, agave syrup, or maple syrup

Instructions:

1. In a jaYog a tall glass, layer the Greek yogurt, granola or crushed nuts, and fresh berries or sliced fruit.

2. Repeat the layers until the jar or glass is filled.

3. Drizzle with honey, agave syrup, or maple syrup if desired.

4. When ready to eat, serve right away or store in the refrigerator.

Benefits: Greek yogurt is a great source of protein, calcium, and probiotics, promoting a healthy digestive system. The addition of berries provides antioxidants and essential vitamins.

4. Veggie Omelette:

Ingredients:

- 2–3 large eggs

- Assorted vegetables (spinach, bell peppers, onions, mushrooms, etc.)

- Salt, pepper, and herbs/spices of choice

- Olive oil or cooking spray

Instructions:

1. Chop the assorted vegetables into small pieces.

2. In a bowl, whisk the eggs until well combined. Add salt, pepper, and herbs/spices of your choice.

3. Heat olive oil or cooking spray in a skillet over medium heat.

4. Add the chopped vegetables and sauté until they are cooked to your desired tenderness.

5. Evenly cover the veggies with the whisked eggs.

6. Cook the omelette for a few minutes until the eggs are set.

7. Flip one half of the omelet onto the other half and let it cook for another minute or two.

8. Slide the omelet onto a plate and serve hot.

Benefits: This protein-packed omelet is an excellent way to incorporate vegetables into your breakfast, providing essential nutrients and a balanced start to your day.

Conclusion:

With these quick and easy breakfast recipes, you can ensure a nutritious and satisfying start to your day without compromising on time. These recipes are versatile, allowing you to customize them according to your preferences and dietary needs. By incorporating these ideas into your morning routine, you can prioritize your overall well-being and fuel your body and mind for a productive day ahead.

Chapter 6. Lunch and Dinner Ideas for Diabetes

In order to effectively control blood sugar levels, people with diabetes must maintain a healthy diet. Choosing the right foods and incorporating balanced meals is crucial for providing energy and essential nutrients while keeping blood sugar levels stable. Here are some comprehensive lunch and dinner ideas that are delicious, nutritiously balanced, and suitable for individuals with diabetes.

Lunch Ideas:

1. Grilled Chicken Salad:

- Grilled chicken breast

- Mixed greens (spinach, lettuce, or arugula)

- A variety of veggies, including bell peppers, cucumbers, and cherry tomatoes
- Optional toppings: feta cheese, nuts, seeds
- Thoroughly coat the salad with the dressing just before serving.

Instructions:

- Toss the mixed greens and vegetables in a bowl.
- Grill the chicken breast until cooked through, then slice into strips.
- Add the chicken to the salad.
- Top with optional toppings.
- Thoroughly coat the salad with the dressing just before serving.

Benefits: This salad provides lean protein from the chicken, fiber from the vegetables, and healthy fats from the olive oil. It is low in carbs and ideal for maintaining stable blood sugar levels.

2. Quinoa and Vegetable Stir-Fry:
- Cooked quinoa (portion control based on dietary needs)
- A variety of veggies, such as snap peas, bell peppers, and broccoli
- Garlic and ginger (minced)
- Low-sodium soy sauce or tamari

Instructions:
- Heat a tablespoon of olive oil in a skillet or wok.
- Stir-fry the ginger and garlic until aromatic.
- Add the assortment of vegetables and sauté until they reach desired tenderness.
- Mix in the cooked quinoa.
- Use tamari or low-sodium soy sauce for seasoning.

- Toss everything together until well combined.

Benefits: Quinoa is a low-glycemic index grain, providing steady energy without spiking blood sugar levels. Vegetables are rich in fiber, vitamins, and minerals, making this dish an ideal choice for blood glucose control.

Dinner Ideas:

1. Baked Salmon with Roasted Vegetables:
- Salmon fillet
- Assorted vegetables (asparagus, carrots, Brussels sprouts)
- Olive oil
- Lemon juice
- Garlic powder, salt, and pepper

Instructions:
- Preheat the oven to 400°F (200°C).

- Arrange the salmon fillet on a parchment paper-lined baking sheet.
- Pour lemon juice and olive oil onto the salmon.
- Season with garlic powder, salt, and pepper.
- Toss the assorted vegetables in olive oil, salt, and pepper on another baking sheet.
- Bake the salmon and vegetables for about 15-20 minutes, or until the salmon is cooked through and the vegetables are roasted to perfection.

Benefits: Salmon is an excellent source of omega-3 fatty acids, which can help reduce inflammation and lower the risk of heart disease. Roasted vegetables provide fiber and essential nutrients, making this a nourishing and blood sugar-friendly dinner option.

2. Turkey Chili:

- Lean ground turkey

- Onion (diced)

- Assorted bell peppers (diced)

- Canned crushed tomatoes (no added sugar)

- Kidney beans (rinsed and drained)

- Chili powder, cumin, paprika, salt, and pepper (to taste)

Instructions:

- In a large pot, cook the ground turkey until browned.

- Add the diced onion and bell peppers and sauté until softened.

- Stir in the crushed tomatoes and kidney beans.

- Add salt, pepper, cumin, paprika, and chili powder for seasoning.

- Simmer on low heat for about 30 minutes, allowing the flavors to meld together.
- Serve hot garnished with fresh herbs, such as cilantro or parsley.

Benefits: Turkey is a lean source of protein, and the combination of vegetables and beans in chili provides fiber and essential nutrients. This low-glycemic index meal is satisfying and helps regulate blood sugar levels.

Conclusion:

When planning meals for individuals with diabetes, it is crucial to choose balanced options that incorporate lean proteins, whole grains, fiber-rich vegetables, and healthy fats. The lunch and dinner ideas mentioned above are delicious, diabetes-friendly choices that help maintain stable blood sugar levels while providing essential nutrients and satisfying meals. Remember to consult with a healthcare professional or a registered dietitian for personalized recommendations based on your specific dietary needs and diabetes management plan.

Balanced Meal Options with Diabetes-Friendly Ingredients

It's critical for people with diabetes to maintain a healthy, balanced diet. By incorporating diabetes-friendly ingredients into meals, one can effectively manage blood sugar levels, promote overall well-being, and reduce the risk of complications. In this comprehensive note, we will explore various components of a balanced meal and suggest diabetes-friendly ingredients for each category.

1. Complex Carbohydrates:

Diabetes-friendly complex carbohydrates help regulate blood sugar levels and provide essential nutrients. Some great options include:

- Whole grains include pasta, whole wheat bread, quinoa, brown rice, and oats.

- Legumes: kidney, black, chickpeas, and lentils.

- Non-starchy vegetables: bell peppers, zucchini, cauliflower, broccoli, and spinach.

2. Lean Proteins:

Including lean proteins in meals helps maintain muscle mass, promotes satiety, and stabilizes blood sugar levels. Opt for:

- Skinless poultry: chicken breast, turkey breast.
- Fish: salmon, tuna, sardines, and trout.
- Plant-based proteins: tofu, tempeh, and legumes (mentioned above).

3. Healthy Fats:

Incorporating healthy fats into meals aids in managing blood sugar levels and provides essential nutrients. Diabetes-friendly fat options include:

- Avocado: packed with heart-healthy monounsaturated fats.
- Seeds and nuts: flaxseeds, chia seeds, walnuts, and almonds.
- Olive oil: a great choice for cooking and dressings.

- Fatty fish: salmon and mackerel, rich in omega-3 fatty acids.

4. Non-Starchy Vegetables:

Non-starchy vegetables are low in carbohydrates and high in fiber, making them excellent choices for people with diabetes. Some examples are:

- Greens that are leafy, such as kale, spinach, and Swiss chard.

- Cruciferous vegetables: broccoli, cauliflower, Brussels sprouts, and cabbage.

- Tomatoes, cucumber, bell peppers, and mushrooms.

5. Portion Control:

Maintaining portion control is essential for controlling blood sugar levels. Using measuring tools, such as cups and scales, can help ensure appropriate serving sizes.

It's also important to balance the types of foods on the plate by including appropriate proportions of carbohydrates, proteins, and fats.

6. Beverage Choices:
Diabetes-friendly beverage options help maintain hydration without raising blood sugar levels. Examples include:
- Water: the best hydrating choice.
- Unsweetened tea: green, herbal, or black tea.
- Sugar-free and unsweetened drinks.

Conclusion:
Incorporating diabetes-friendly ingredients into a balanced meal is crucial for individuals with diabetes to manage their blood sugar levels effectively. By focusing on complex carbohydrates, lean proteins, healthy fats, non-starchy

vegetables, portion control, and diabetes-friendly beverages, one can create a variety of delicious meals that promote overall health and wellbeing. Remember to consult a healthcare professional or registered dietitian for personalized advice and guidance based on your individual needs.

Recipes for Nutritious Lunch and Dinner Meals

Preparing nutritious lunch and dinner meals is essential for maintaining a healthy lifestyle. By incorporating a variety of wholesome ingredients, one can create meals that are both delicious and nourishing. In this comprehensive note, we will explore some recipe ideas for nutritious lunch and dinner meals, focusing on balanced combinations of macronutrients and diabetes-friendly options.

1. Grilled Chicken Salad:

Ingredients:

- Grilled chicken breast (lean protein)
- Mixed greens, such as spinach, lettuce, and arugula (non-starchy vegetables)
- Cherry tomatoes (non-starchy vegetables)
- Cucumbers (non-starchy vegetables)
- Avocado slices (healthy fats)
- Olive oil and vinegar dressing (healthy fats)

Instructions:

1. Season and grill the chicken breast until cooked thoroughly.
2. In a large bowl, combine the mixed greens, cherry tomatoes, and cucumbers.

3. Slice the grilled chicken and place it on top of the salad.

4. Add avocado slices and drizzle with olive oil and vinegar dressing.

2. Baked Salmon with Quinoa and Roasted Vegetables:

Ingredients:

- Salmon fillet (lean protein)

- Quinoa (complex carbohydrates)

- Assorted vegetables, such as broccoli, bell peppers, and zucchini (non-starchy vegetables)

- Olive oil (healthy fats)

Instructions:

1. Set the oven's temperature to your preferred setting.

2. Season the salmon with salt, pepper, and any desired herbs or spices.

3. Place the salmon on a baking sheet and bake until cooked.

4. Cook quinoa according to package instructions.

5. Toss the assorted vegetables in olive oil, salt, and pepper, then roast in the oven until tender.

6. Serve the baked salmon with quinoa and roasted vegetables.

3. Stir-Fried Tofu with Brown Rice and Steamed Vegetables:
Ingredients:
- Firm tofu (plant-based protein)
- Brown rice (complex carbohydrates)
- Assorted vegetables, such as broccoli, carrots, and snow peas (non-starchy vegetables)
- Low-sodium soy sauce or tamari (low-sodium flavoring)

Instructions:

1. Drain and press tofu to remove excess moisture, then cut into cubes.

2. Cook brown rice according to package instructions.

3. In a pan or wok, heat a small amount of oil and stir-fry the tofu until golden.

4. Add the assorted vegetables and continue to stir-fry until just cooked.

5. Season with low-sodium soy sauce or tamari.

6. Serve the stir-fried tofu and vegetables over a bed of brown rice.

Conclusion:

Preparing nutritious lunch and dinner meals is essential for maintaining a well-balanced diet. The recipes mentioned above provide a combination of lean proteins, complex carbohydrates, non-starchy vegetables, and healthy fats.

Remember to personalize these recipes according to your dietary needs and preferences. Additionally, consult a healthcare professional or registered dietitian for personalized advice and guidance based on your specific requirements.

Chapter 7. Snacks and Desserts for Diabetes

Snacks and desserts can be an enjoyable part of a healthy, balanced diet for individuals with diabetes. With careful planning and moderation, it is possible to indulge in delicious treats without compromising blood sugar levels. Here are some guidelines and ideas for snacks and desserts that are suitable for individuals managing diabetes:

1. Focus on nutrient-dense options: Opt for snacks and desserts that provide important nutrients while keeping carbohydrates and added sugars in check. This ensures stable blood sugar levels and overall good health.

2. Portion control is key: Regardless of the snack or dessert, portion control is crucial for managing diabetes. Pay attention to serving sizes and avoid mindless snacking, as excess consumption can affect blood sugar levels.

3. Include protein and fiber: Protein and fiber help slow down the absorption of glucose, promoting better blood sugar control. Incorporate these nutrients into your snacks and desserts to increase satiety and regulate blood sugar levels.

4. Choose whole foods: Whole foods are minimally processed and contain more fiber, vitamins, and minerals. Incorporating whole foods like fruits, vegetables, nuts, and seeds into your snacks and desserts can provide a healthier alternative to processed options.

5. Be mindful of carbohydrates: Carbohydrate counting is a typical part of diabetes management. When selecting snacks and desserts, consider the carbohydrate content and choose those that fit within your overall carbohydrate intake goals.

Snack Ideas:
- Apple slices with almond butter
- Greek yogurt with mixed berries
- Celery sticks with hummus
- Hard-boiled eggs
- Mixed nuts (portion-controlled)
- Baby carrots with guacamole
- Sugar-free, whole grain cereal with low-fat milk
- Air-popped popcorn (lightly salted)

Dessert Ideas:

- Mixed fruit salad with a sprinkle of cinnamon
- Greek yogurt parfait with fresh berries and a drizzle of honey (in moderation)
- Baked apple slices with a sprinkle of cinnamon and a dollop of unsweetened whipped cream
- Chia seed pudding made with unsweetened almond milk and topped with diced fruits
- Dark chocolate (70% cocoa or more) with a few almonds
- Sugar-free, homemade fruit sorbet
- Mini oatmeal cookies made with whole grain oats and a sugar substitute

Remember, it is important to consult with a healthcare professional or registered dietitian for personalized advice on managing diabetes and incorporating snacks and desserts into your specific meal plan.

Healthy Snack Choices for Blood Sugar Control

Maintaining stable blood sugar levels is important for overall health, particularly for individuals with diabetes or pre-diabetes. Making smart snacking choices is essential to prevent blood sugar spikes and crashes throughout the day. This comprehensive note aims to provide you with helpful tips and a list of healthy snack choices to incorporate into your diet for optimal blood sugar control.

Tips for Blood Sugar Control:

1. Choose Fiber-rich Foods: Opt for snacks that are high in dietary fiber as they can help slow down the absorption of glucose into the bloodstream, thus preventing sudden spikes in blood sugar levels.

2. Include Protein: Protein-rich snacks can help increase satiety, regulate blood sugar levels, and promote healthy weight management. Combining protein with carbohydrates can also slow down the digestion and absorption of sugars.

3. Mindful Portion Control: Even healthy snacks can affect blood sugar levels if consumed in large quantities. Pay attention to portion sizes and refrain from mindless snacking.

4. Avoid Refined Carbohydrates and Added Sugars: Snacks high in refined carbohydrates and added sugars can cause rapid spikes in blood sugar levels. Choose snacks with natural sugars and complex carbohydrates instead.

5. Combine Foods Effectively: Pairing carbohydrates with healthy fats or proteins can help slow down the release of glucose into the bloodstream. This can aid in better blood sugar management.

Healthy Snack Choices:

1. Nuts and Seeds: Almonds, walnuts, chia seeds, flaxseeds, and pumpkin seeds are excellent sources of healthy fats, fiber, and protein. They provide energy, promote satiety, and stabilize blood sugar levels.

2. Greek Yogurt: Low-fat Greek yogurt is high in protein and low in carbohydrates. It makes for a satisfying snack on its own or can be combined with nuts, seeds, or berries for added nutrition and flavor.

3. Fresh Fruits and Veggies: Choose non-starchy vegetables such as carrots, celery sticks, bell peppers, and cherry tomatoes. Fruits like berries, apples, and oranges are rich in fiber, antioxidants, and natural sugars.

4. Hummus and Veggie Sticks: Opt for hummus as a dip and accompany it with cut-up vegetables like cucumbers, celery, and bell peppers. Hummus is high in protein and fiber, making it an ideal blood sugar-friendly snack.

5. Hard-Boiled Eggs: Eggs are an excellent source of protein and healthy fats. Hard-boiled eggs make for a quick and convenient snack option. Pair them with a side of vegetable sticks for added nutrients.

6. Whole Grain Crackers or Rice Cakes: Look for whole grain options that are low in added sugars and high in fiber. Pair with toppings such as avocado, nut butter, or low-fat cheese for added flavor and satiety.

7. Cottage Cheese: Cottage cheese is low in carbohydrates and high in protein. It can be enjoyed plain or topped with fresh fruits or a sprinkle of cinnamon for added taste.

Conclusion:

When it comes to blood sugar control, making smart snack choices is crucial. By incorporating fiber-rich foods, protein sources, and mindful portion control, you can maintain stable blood sugar levels throughout the day. Experiment with the suggested snack choices above to find the ones that suit your taste and dietary needs. Remember to consult a healthcare professional or registered dietitian for personalized guidance on managing your blood sugar levels

Sugar-Free Dessert Alternatives

For individuals looking to reduce their sugar intake or manage conditions like diabetes, finding sugar-free dessert options can be a challenge. Thankfully, there are numerous delicious alternatives available that satisfy cravings without compromising taste. This comprehensive note explores various sugar-free dessert alternatives that can be incorporated into a balanced diet.

Tips for Choosing Sugar-Free Desserts:

1. Natural Sweeteners: Look for desserts sweetened with natural alternatives like stevia, erythritol, monk fruit extract, or xylitol. These options provide sweetness without causing spikes in blood sugar levels.

2. Fruits: Incorporate fresh or frozen fruits into desserts for natural sweetness. Fruits like berries, apples, and citrus fruits add flavor, fiber, and essential nutrients.

3. Sugar Substitutes: Experiment with sugar substitutes like sucralose or aspartame. While these artificial sweeteners lack calories and do not raise blood sugar levels, it is important to consume them in moderation.

4. Healthy Fats: Incorporate ingredients rich in healthy fats like avocados, nuts, and seeds. These ingredients add texture and satiety to desserts while promoting a feeling of fullness.

5. Portion Control: Even sugar-free desserts should be consumed in moderation. Pay attention to portion sizes and enjoy desserts as part of a balanced diet.

Sugar-Free Dessert Alternatives:

1. Fresh Fruit Salad: Create a colorful fruit salad with a mixture of berries, sliced apples, oranges, and melons. For added flavor, sprinkle with a squeeze of lemon juice or a dash of cinnamon.

2. **Chia Pudding**: Mix chia seeds with unsweetened almond or coconut milk, and sweeten with a natural sweetener or a few drops of vanilla extract. Refrigerate the mixture overnight to allow it to thicken. Top with fresh berries or chopped nuts for extra texture.

3. **Sugar-Free Gelatin**: Enjoy a light and refreshing dessert by making sugar-free gelatin using a sugar-free gelatin mix and water. Mix in fresh fruit pieces before refrigerating for a fun twist.

4. **Greek Yogurt Parfait**: Layer low-fat or non-fat Greek yogurt with fresh berries and a sprinkle of chopped nuts or seeds. Add a drizzle of sugar-free syrup for added sweetness if desired.

5. Avocado Chocolate Mousse: Blend ripe avocados, unsweetened cocoa powder, a natural sweetener, and a splash of vanilla extract until smooth and creamy. Chill in the refrigerator and serve topped with a dollop of unsweetened whipped cream or fresh berries.

6. Baked Fruit Crumble: Mix together a mixture of oats, almond flour, cinnamon, and a natural sweetener. Sprinkle the mixture on top of sliced apples, pears, or berries, and bake until golden and bubbly.

7. Frozen Yogurt Popsicles: Blend plain Greek yogurt with a natural sweetener, fruit puree, and a touch of vanilla extract. Pour into popsicle molds and freeze for a refreshing and guilt-free treat.

Conclusion:

Enjoying sugar-free desserts doesn't mean sacrificing taste or pleasure. With a bit of creativity and the incorporation of natural sweeteners, fruits, and healthy fats, you can indulge in delicious treats while maintaining a balanced diet. Remember to consume these desserts in moderation and consult with a healthcare professional or registered dietitian if you have specific dietary needs or concerns.

Delicious Snack and Dessert Recipes

Exploring new recipes and trying out delicious snacks and desserts can be a delightful way to satisfy cravings and enjoy treats. This comprehensive note provides a collection of mouthwatering recipes for both snacks and desserts that you can enjoy with family and friends.

1. Energy Boosting Snacks:

a) No-Bake Energy Bites:

Ingredients:

- 1 cup rolled oats

- 1/2 cup nut butter

- 1/4 cup honey or maple syrup

- 1/4 cup ground flaxseed

- 1/4 cup mini chocolate chips

- 1 tsp vanilla extract

Instructions:

Thoroughly combine all the ingredients in a mixing bowl. Form the mixture into tiny balls that are bite-sized. To set, put them in the fridge for thirty minutes. Enjoy as a speedy and wholesome snack.

b) Mini Quiches with Stuffed Veggies:
Components:

- Six big eggs

1-/4 cup of milk

- 1/2 cup of finely chopped veggies, such as spinach, onions, and bell peppers.

– 1/4 cup of cheese, shredded

To taste, add salt and pepper.

Guidelines:

Set a muffin tin to 375°F (190°C) and preheat the oven. Turn the milk and eggs together in a bowl. Add the cheese, chopped veggies, salt, and pepper and stir. Fill each cup of the muffin tin about 3/4 of the way to the top with the mixture. Bake until set and slightly golden, 15 to 20 minutes. Let cool slightly before taking them out of the tin. Serve warm or cold.

2. Decadent Dessert Recipes:

a) Flourless Chocolate Cake:

Ingredients:

- 8 oz dark chocolate, chopped

- 1/2 cup unsalted butter

- 3/4 cup of powdered sugar or a different type of sweetener

- 4 large eggs

- 1 tsp vanilla extract

- Pinch of salt

- Cocoa powder for dusting (optional)

Instructions:

Preheat the oven to 350°F (175°C) and grease a round cake pan. Place the chocolate and butter in a microwave-safe bowl and melt in short intervals, stirring until smooth. In a separate bowl, whisk together the sugar, eggs, vanilla extract, and salt. Gradually add the melted chocolate mixture to the whisked ingredients and combine well. Pour the batter into the prepared pan and bake for 25-30 minutes until the center is set. When taking the cake out of the pan, let it cool. If desired, sprinkle with cocoa powder.

b) Fruit Parfait Fresh:

Components:

- One cup of yogurt

- One cup of mixed fresh berries, including raspberries, blueberries, and strawberries

- 1/4 cup of granola or crushed nuts

- Optional: honey or maple syrup

Instructions: Arrange the Greek yogurt, nuts or granola, and fresh berries in a glass or jar. Until all of the ingredients are used, keep layering. Drizzle honey or maple syrup on top for added sweetness if desired. Serve chilled.

Conclusion:

These snack and dessert recipes provide a variety of options to satisfy your cravings and enjoy delightful treats. Whether you're in the mood for a quick energy boost or a decadent dessert, these recipes are sure to please your taste buds. Remember to adjust the recipes to your dietary preferences or consult a healthcare professional or registered dietitian for personalized guidance. Enjoy creating and indulging in these delicious snacks and desserts!

Chapter 8. Beverages for Diabetes

A metabolic disease called diabetes is typified by elevated blood sugar levels. When managing diabetes, people need to be cautious about their dietary choices, including their beverage intake. This comprehensive note aims to provide valuable information on selecting suitable beverages for individuals with diabetes to help maintain blood sugar control and overall health.

General Guidelines for Beverage Choices:

1. Stay Hydrated: Adequate hydration is essential for everyone, including people with diabetes. Opt for calorie-free and sugar-free options like water and unsweetened tea as your primary sources of hydration.

2. Portion Control: Carefully manage portion sizes, as excessive consumption of any beverage, even those without sugar, can impact blood sugar levels and overall calorie intake.

Beverage Recommendations:

1. Water: No calories, no sugar, and unmatched hydration properties make water the preferred beverage for people with diabetes. Stay well-hydrated by consuming plain or infused water throughout the day.

2. Tea:

a. Green tea: It contains no calories and is high in antioxidants, which may help manage blood sugar levels and improve insulin sensitivity.

b. Herbal tea: Herbal teas like chamomile, peppermint, or cinnamon can be enjoyed without sugar and may have additional health benefits, like promoting relaxation or reducing inflammation.

3. Coffee:

a. **Black coffee**: Enjoying plain black coffee (without sugar or cream) in moderation is generally considered safe for people with diabetes. However, note that caffeine can affect blood sugar levels differently for each individual, so monitor your response.

b. **Avoid sugary coffee beverages**: Steer clear of coffee drinks loaded with sugar, syrups, whipped cream, or flavored creamers, as they can rapidly increase blood sugar levels.

4. Low-fat milk and dairy alternatives:

a. **Skim or low-fat milk**: Low in fat and carbohydrates, skim or low-fat milk can be a good source of calcium and protein. However, it's important to consider the carbohydrate content and portion sizes while incorporating it into your meal plan.

b. Dairy alternatives: Unsweetened almond milk, soy milk, or coconut milk (without added sugars) are viable options for those who are lactose intolerant or prefer plant-based alternatives. Choose the unsweetened versions to minimize carbohydrate intake.

5. Sparkling water/Club soda: Unsweetened sparkling water or club soda can be a refreshing and tasty alternative to sugary carbonated drinks. Ensure you check the label to confirm there are no added sugars or sweeteners.

6. Vegetable Juice:

a. Tomato juice: With a lower sugar content compared to fruit juices, unsalted tomato juice can be enjoyed in moderation.

b. Homemade vegetable juice: By blending fresh vegetables like spinach, kale, cucumber, and celery, you can create a nutrient-rich beverage without added sugars.

7. Smoothies:

a. Homemade smoothies: Prepare your own smoothies using low-sugar fruits (e.g., berries), leafy greens, and low-fat yogurt. Monitor your portion sizes and adjust the ingredients based on your meal plan and blood sugar control.

b. Be mindful of sugary additives: Avoid adding sugar, honey, or syrups to your smoothies and be cautious of store-bought smoothies, which often contain added sugars.

Conclusion:

Choosing appropriate beverages is crucial for managing diabetes effectively. Focus on hydration, portion control, and selecting options without added sugars and excess carbohydrates. Incorporating water, unsweetened tea, coffee (in moderation), low-fat milk or dairy alternatives, vegetable juice, sparkling water, and homemade smoothies can provide variety while prioritizing blood sugar control and overall health. Remember to consult with a healthcare professional or registered dietitian for personalized guidance based on your specific dietary needs and diabetes management goals.

Best Drink Choices to Maintain Stable Blood Sugar Levels

Maintaining stable blood sugar levels is crucial for individuals with diabetes, as it helps promote overall health and prevents complications. Proper beverage selection plays a vital role in managing blood sugar levels. This comprehensive note aims to provide valuable information on the best drink choices to help maintain stable blood sugar levels.

General Guidelines for Beverage Choices:

1. **Choose Hydrating Options:** Adequate hydration is essential for everyone, including individuals with diabetes. Opt for calorie-free and sugar-free options as your primary sources of hydration.

2. **Portion Control**: Be mindful of portion sizes, as excessive consumption of any beverage, even those without added sugars, can impact blood sugar levels.

Best Drink Choices to Maintain Stable Blood Sugar Levels:

1. **Water**: Water is the ultimate drink choice for maintaining stable blood sugar levels. It contains no calories, no sugar, and is essential for optimal hydration. Aim to drink an adequate amount of plain or infused water throughout the day to stay hydrated.

2. **Herbal Tea**: Herbal teas offer a variety of flavors and health benefits without adding extra sugar or calories. Consider choosing herbal teas such as chamomile, peppermint, ginger, or cinnamon. These teas are known to provide relaxation, aid digestion, and potentially help regulate blood sugar levels.

3. **Green Tea**: Green tea is rich in antioxidants and has been shown to have some potential benefits for individuals with diabetes. It might support better insulin sensitivity and blood sugar

regulation. Opt for unsweetened green tea for the best results.

4. Unsweetened Coffee: Enjoying black coffee without sugar or cream in moderation is generally considered safe for people with diabetes. However, individual responses to caffeine may vary, so it's essential to monitor blood sugar levels. Adding excessive sugar or consuming specialty coffee beverages high in added sugars should be avoided.

5. Caffeine-free Herbal Coffee Alternatives: Some caffeine-free herbal coffee substitutes, such as roasted chicory root or dandelion tea, can be a suitable option for individuals avoiding caffeine. Just ensure these alternatives are unsweetened and do not contain added sugars.

6. Low-Fat Milk and Dairy Alternatives: Low-fat milk and unsweetened dairy alternatives like almond milk or soy milk can be consumed in moderation. They provide essential nutrients like calcium and protein. However, it's important to be mindful of portion sizes and consider the carbohydrate content as part of your meal plan.

7. Sparkling Water/Club Soda: Unsweetened sparkling water or club soda can provide a refreshing carbonated beverage option without adding extra sugar or calories. These can be a great alternative to sugary carbonated drinks.

8. Fruit Infused Water: Adding slices of fruits like lemon, lime, or cucumber to your water can provide a hint of flavor without adding excessive sugar or calories. Experiment with different combinations of fruits and herbs to enjoy a refreshing infusion.

9. Vegetable Juice: Homemade vegetable juices made from fresh vegetables are an excellent choice for individuals with diabetes. However, it is important to monitor portion sizes and consider the carbohydrate content as some vegetable juices can contain higher amounts of natural sugars.

10. Homemade Smoothies: Creating your own smoothies using low-sugar fruits (e.g., berries), leafy greens, and unsweetened yogurt or milk alternatives can provide a nutrient-rich beverage option. Be cautious of the portion sizes and avoid adding extra sugars or sweeteners.

Conclusion:Selecting the best drink choices is crucial for maintaining stable blood sugar levels for individuals with diabetes. Focus on hydrating options like water, herbal tea, and unsweetened coffee. Incorporate low-fat milk or dairy alternatives in moderation. Sparkling water can provide a refreshing carbonated drink alternative. Experiment with fruit-infused water, vegetable juices, and homemade smoothies while being mindful of portion sizes and carbohydrate content. It is always prudent to consult with a healthcare professional or registered dietitian for personalized guidance based on individual dietary needs and diabetes management goals.

Diabetes-Friendly Beverage Recipes

Diabetes-friendly beverage recipes can be a great way to enjoy flavorful and refreshing drinks while keeping blood sugar levels in check. This comprehensive note provides a selection of delicious, diabetes-friendly beverage recipes that incorporate low-sugar, low-carbohydrate ingredients to help maintain stable blood sugar levels.

1. Citrus Infused Water:

Ingredients:

- 1 lemon (sliced)

- 1 lime (sliced)

- 1 orange (sliced)

- Mint leaves (optional)

- Ice cubes

- Water

Instructions:

1. Place the sliced citrus fruits and mint leaves (if desired) in a pitcher.

2. Fill the pitcher with water and add ice cubes.

3. Stir gently to combine the flavors.

4. Give the mixture at least an hour to infuse in the refrigerator.

5. Serve chilled and enjoy the refreshing and naturally sweetened citrus-infused water.

2. Cucumber Mint Cooler:

Ingredients:

- 1 cucumber (peeled and sliced)

- 10-12 fresh mint leaves

- Juice of 1 lime

- 2 cups of water

- Ice cubes

Instructions:

1. In a blender, combine the cucumber slices, mint leaves, lime juice, and water.

2. Blend until smooth.

3. Strain the mixture to remove any pulp (optional).

4. Fill glasses with ice cubes and pour the cucumber mint cooler over the ice.

5. Add a sprig of mint as a garnish and stir gently.

6. Serve cold as a revitalizing and răcorous drink.

3. Chia Seed Smoothie with Berries:

Ingredients:

- One cup of berries, including strawberries, blueberries, and raspberries. One-third cup chia seeds

- One cup of plain almond milk (or any other type of milk substitute)

- 1-2 teaspoons of stevia or another sugar substitute (optional)

- Ice cubes (optional)

Instructions:

1. In a blender, combine the mixed berries, chia seeds, almond milk, and stevia (if desired).

2. Blend until smooth.

3. Add ice cubes if a colder consistency is desired.

4. Pour into glasses and serve chilled.

4. Iced Green Tea with Lemon:

Ingredients:

- 2 green tea bags

- 4 cups water

- Juice of 1 lemon

- Ice cubes

Instructions:

1. Heat some water in a pot until it boils.

2. Remove the pot from heat and add the green tea bags.

3. Allow the tea bags to steep for 3-5 minutes.

4. Remove the tea bags and let the tea cool to room temperature.

5. Add the lemon juice to the cooled tea and stir well.

6. Pour the tea into a pitcher and refrigerate until chilled.

7. Serve over ice cubes as a refreshing and diabetes-friendly iced tea.

5. Spiced Apple Cider:

Ingredients:

- 2 cups unsweetened apple juice

- 2 cups water

- 2 cinnamon sticks

- 2-3 whole cloves

- 1-2 teaspoons of stevia or another sugar substitute (optional)

Instructions:

1. In a pot, combine the apple juice, water, cinnamon sticks, cloves, and stevia (if desired).

2. Bring the mixture to a simmer over low heat for about 10 minutes.

3. Remove the pot from heat and strain the spiced apple cider into mugs.

4. Serve warm and enjoy the comforting flavors of this diabetes-friendly beverage.

Conclusion:

These diabetes-friendly beverage recipes offer a range of refreshing and flavorful options that are low in sugar and carbohydrates. Whether you prefer infused water, coolers, smoothies, or warm beverages, these recipes provide alternatives that help maintain stable blood sugar levels without compromising taste. Remember to consult with a healthcare professional or registered dietitian to tailor these recipes to your individual dietary needs and diabetes management goals. Enjoy these beverages as part of a well-balanced meal plan and a healthy lifestyle.

Chapter 9. Eating Out with Diabetes

Managing diabetes requires careful attention to lifestyle choices, including dietary habits. However, enjoying a meal out at a restaurant with friends, family, or colleagues doesn't have to be a daunting task if you have diabetes. With a little planning and knowledge, you can still savor delicious meals while maintaining stable blood sugar levels. Here are some tips to help you navigate eating out with diabetes:

1. Choose the Right Restaurant: Selecting the right restaurant can make a significant difference in managing your diabetes. Look for establishments that offer healthy options, such as those with a variety of vegetables, lean proteins, and whole grains on their menu. Websites and mobile applications that provide nutrition information and user reviews can be helpful resources in making informed decisions.

2. Plan Ahead: If possible, review the menu and make choices ahead of time. Many restaurants now provide their menus online, allowing you to analyze nutritional information and plan your meal accordingly. This can help you make healthier choices and avoid impulsive decisions at the restaurant.

3. Watch Portion Sizes: Restaurants often serve generous portions, so be mindful of portion sizes. Consider splitting a dish with a companion or ask the waitstaff to pack half of your meal to take home before it is served. This will help you maintain better control over portion sizes and avoid overeating.

4. Control Carbohydrate Intake: Monitor your carbohydrate consumption, as it plays a major role in blood sugar management. Choose whole-grain options, such as brown rice or whole-wheat bread, instead of refined grains. When ordering pasta, consider opting for whole wheat or alternative grain options like quinoa or lentil pasta. Additionally, aim to include a source of lean protein, such as chicken, fish, tofu, or legumes, with your meal to help slow down carbohydrate absorption.

5. Take Control of Preparation Methods: Request that your food be prepared using healthier cooking techniques, such as grilling, baking, steaming, or broiling, instead of frying. Ask for sauces, dressings, and condiments to be served on the side so that you can control the amount used, as these often contain hidden sugars and unhealthy fats.

6. Stay Hydrated: Drink water with your meal instead of sugary beverages like soda or sweetened juices. If you prefer something more flavorful, ask for water infused with lemon, lime, or cucumber. Be cautious of alcoholic drinks, as they can significantly impact blood sugar levels. If you choose to consume alcohol, do so in moderation, and always consult with your healthcare team regarding alcohol consumption and medication interactions.

7. Inform the Waitstaff: Let your server know about your dietary needs and restrictions, including your diabetes. They can often provide recommendations or accommodate specific requests, such as substituting certain ingredients or altering cooking methods. Don't hesitate to ask questions about the menu or any concerns you may have.

8. Be Mindful of Desserts: While desserts can be tempting, try to opt for healthier alternatives, such as fresh fruit, yogurt, or a small portion of sugar-free options. If you choose to indulge in a sweet treat, consider sharing it with someone or saving it for another occasion.

Remember, maintaining a balanced diet and managing blood sugar levels is crucial for diabetes management. By planning ahead, making smart menu choices, and being conscious of portion sizes and preparation methods, you can still enjoy dining out while keeping your diabetes under control. It's always advisable to consult with your healthcare team for personalized advice and recommendations.

Tips for Making Healthy Choices at Restaurants

Eating out at restaurants can be enjoyable and convenient, but it can also present challenges when it comes to making healthy choices. However, with some awareness and proactive decision-making, it is possible to enjoy a restaurant meal while still prioritizing your health and nutrition goals. Here are some tips for making healthy choices at restaurants:

1. **Research and Choose Wisely**: Before heading out, take the time to research restaurants in your area that offer healthier options. Many establishments now provide nutritional information on their websites or through mobile apps, which can guide your decision-making process. Look for menus that include a variety of vegetables, lean proteins, whole grains, and healthier cooking methods.

2. **Control Portion Sizes**: Restaurant portions are often larger than what you would typically consume at home. To avoid overeating, try splitting a meal with a dining companion or request a to-go box at the beginning of the meal and save half for later. Alternatively, you can order an appetizer or side dish as your main course, as these portions tend to be more reasonable.

3. Start with Soup or Salad: Beginning your meal with a broth-based soup or a side salad can help fill you up on low-calorie, nutrient-dense foods. Opt for clear soups and vinaigrette dressings instead of creamy or high-fat options. This can help control your appetite and reduce the likelihood of overeating during the main course.

4. Customize Your Order: Don't hesitate to ask the waitstaff to customize your order to suit your dietary preferences and needs. Requesting steamed or grilled preparations instead of fried options, substituting high-calorie sides with vegetables or a side salad, or asking for sauces and dressings on the side are all ways to make your meal healthier.

5. Be Mindful of Hidden Ingredients: Some ingredients used in restaurant cooking, such as butter, high-sodium sauces, and added sugars, can significantly impact the nutritional content of your meal. Ask about ingredients or cooking methods if you have any concerns. Opting for dishes that are grilled, baked, or steamed can often be a healthier choice than fried or sautéed options.

6. **Balance Your Plate**: Aim to have a balanced meal that includes a source of lean protein, such as grilled chicken, fish, legumes, or tofu, paired with whole grains and an assortment of vegetables. Choose whole-grain bread, brown rice, or quinoa as healthier carbohydrate options. Adding vegetables to your main dish or ordering a side of steamed vegetables can increase the fiber content and provide essential nutrients.

7. **Watch Your Beverages**: Be mindful of the calories and added sugars found in

beverages. Opt for water, unsweetened iced tea, or sparkling water as a healthier choice. If you choose an alcoholic beverage, consume it in moderation and, when possible, opt for options with lower sugar content, such as dry wines or spirits mixed with soda water or a sugar-free mixer.

8. Enjoy Desserts in Moderation: Desserts can be a tempting part of dining out, but it's essential to enjoy them in moderation. Consider sharing a dessert with your dining companions or choose healthier alternatives like fresh fruit or a small portion of a lighter dessert, such as a sorbet or a fruit-based option.

Remember, making healthy choices at restaurants is about being mindful and proactive in your decision-making. By doing some research, customizing your order, controlling portion sizes, and balancing your meal, you can enjoy dining out while still prioritizing your health and well-being.

Strategies for Managing Blood Sugar Levels while Dining Out

Maintaining stable blood sugar levels is an essential aspect of managing conditions like diabetes. When dining out at restaurants, it can sometimes be challenging to make choices that support your blood sugar management goals. However, with some strategies and proactive decision-making, you can still enjoy a meal out while keeping your blood sugar levels in check. Here are some strategies for managing blood sugar levels while dining out:

1. Plan Ahead and Research: Before going to a restaurant, take the time to review the menu online if available or call ahead to inquire about the types of dishes they offer. Look for healthier options that are lower in carbohydrates and added sugars. Avoid restaurants that primarily serve fried or heavily processed foods.

2. Focus on Whole Foods: Choose dishes that feature whole, unprocessed foods as the main ingredient. For example, lean proteins like grilled chicken or fish, whole grains such as brown rice or quinoa, and a variety of non-starchy vegetables. These foods provide essential nutrients and tend to have a lower impact on blood sugar levels.

3. Watch Carbohydrate Intake: Pay attention to the carbohydrate content of the dishes you select. While carbohydrates are an important part of a balanced meal, it's crucial to manage portion sizes and include more complex carbohydrates. Opt for whole-grain bread, pasta, or rice, and limit refined grains and high-carbohydrate foods like white bread, white rice, or sugary desserts.

4. **Portion Control**: Restaurant portion sizes are often larger than what you would consume at home. Consider sharing a meal with a dining companion, ordering an appetizer as your main course, or asking the waitstaff to pack half of your meal to take home before it is served. This way, you can consume a more appropriate portion size and avoid overeating.

5. **Mindful Eating**: Take your time when eating and savor each bite. Eating slowly and chewing thoroughly can help you gauge your satiety and prevent overeating. Listen to your body's hunger and fullness

cues to guide your eating pace and portion sizes.

6. Request Modifications: Don't hesitate to ask the restaurant staff if they can accommodate specific modifications to your order. For example, request that sauces, dressings, or condiments be served on the side so that you can control the amount used. Ask for vegetables to be steamed instead of sautéed in butter. Making these small adjustments can help manage both carbohydrate and fat intake.

7. Stay Hydrated: Drink plenty of water before, during, and after the meal. This may help you feel less hungry and fuller. Choose water or unsweetened beverages over sugary sodas or fruit juices. Be cautious with alcohol consumption, as it can affect blood sugar levels. If you choose to drink alcohol, do so in moderation and consider checking your blood sugar levels or adjusting medication dosages as necessary.

8. Monitor Blood Sugar Levels: If you have diabetes or are actively managing your blood sugar levels, continue to monitor and track your readings even when dining out. This will help you gauge the impact of certain meals and adjust your insulin or medication as needed.

Remember, maintaining blood sugar control is a personal and ongoing process. Making thoughtful choices, monitoring portion sizes, and being mindful of your carbohydrate intake while dining out can help you manage blood sugar levels effectively. Work closely with your healthcare team to develop an individualized plan that suits your specific needs and aligns with your

Restaurant Menu Selections for Diabetics

When managing diabetes, making healthy food choices is crucial for maintaining stable blood sugar levels. Dining out at restaurants can pose challenges, as many menu options may be high in unhealthy fats, added sugars, and refined carbohydrates. However, with a little knowledge and strategy, you can navigate restaurant menus and select diabetic-friendly options. Here are some considerations for making restaurant menu selections for diabetics:

1. **Focus on Balanced Meals**: Look for dishes that offer a balance of nutrients, including lean proteins, whole grains, and non-starchy vegetables. Opt for protein sources like grilled chicken, fish, tofu, or legumes and choose whole grains like

quinoa, brown rice, or whole-wheat bread when available. Pair these with plenty of colorful vegetables to maximize the nutritional value of your meal.

2. Limit Added Sugars and Refined Carbohydrates: Avoid dishes that are heavily processed or contain excessive amounts of added sugars. Steer clear of sugar-laden sauces, dressings, and sugary beverages. Be cautious of refined carbohydrates like white bread, pasta, or rice. Instead, choose complex carbohydrates that are higher in fiber and have a lower impact on blood sugar levels.

3. Go for Grilled or Baked Options: Opt for dishes that are grilled, baked, steamed, or broiled instead of fried or sautéed. This helps reduce the added fat content and calorie count of the meal. Additionally, ask the restaurant to prepare your food with minimal oil or butter to further reduce unhealthy fats.

4. Choose Healthy Cooking Methods: Look for menu items that are prepared using healthier cooking methods, which can help minimize the use of unhealthy fats. Examples include dishes that are steamed, poached, roasted, or stir-fried with minimal oil. Avoid items labeled as deep-fried, breaded, or pan-fried, as they tend to be higher in unhealthy fats and calories.

5. Be Mindful of Sauces and Dressings: Many sauces and dressings can be high in added sugars and unhealthy fats. Ask for sauces and dressings to be served on the side so that you can control the amount used. Consider using low-fat or light versions, or opt for vinegar-based dressings or olive oil and vinegar for a healthier alternative.

6. Portion Control: Restaurant portions are often larger than what you need for a well-balanced meal. Practice portion control by splitting a dish with a dining companion or requesting a to-go box at the beginning of the meal to save half for later. This helps manage your calorie intake and prevents overeating.

7. Stay Hydrated with Unsweetened Beverages: Choose water, unsweetened tea, or sparkling water as your beverage options. Steer clear of fruit juices, sugar-filled sodas, and sweetened drinks. If you prefer something a little more flavorful, consider adding a slice of lemon, lime, or cucumber to your water for a refreshing twist.

8. Be Mindful of Dessert Choices: When it comes to desserts, it's important to exercise moderation. Opt for fresh fruit, a small portion of sugar-free options, or share a dessert with others to satisfy your sweet tooth without overindulging.

Remember, everyone's dietary needs are unique, so it's essential to work closely with your healthcare team to develop a personalized meal plan that meets your specific requirements. By being mindful of your food choices, balancing your nutrient intake, and prioritizing whole, unprocessed foods, you can enjoy a delicious meal at a restaurant while managing your diabetes effectively

Chapter 10. Grocery Shopping Tips for Diabetes

When managing diabetes, making well-informed choices while grocery shopping is vital to maintain balanced blood sugar levels and overall health. With proper planning and selection, you can create a nutritious and diabetes-friendly eating plan. This comprehensive note provides valuable grocery shopping tips to help individuals with diabetes make healthier choices and manage their condition more effectively.

1. Plan Ahead:

Before heading to the grocery store, take some time to plan your meals and make a shopping list. This will help you stay focused and avoid impulse purchases that may not align with your dietary needs. Plan a variety of nutrient-rich meals that include whole grains, lean proteins, healthy fats, and plenty of fruits and vegetables.

2. Choose Carbohydrates Wisely:
Carbohydrates have the most significant impact on blood sugar levels, so it's crucial to make smart choices when it comes to carb-containing foods. Opt for complex carbohydrates that have a lower glycemic index, such as whole grains (brown rice, quinoa, whole wheat bread) and legumes (beans, lentils, chickpeas). By releasing glucose more gradually, these foods help to avoid sharp increases in blood sugar levels.

3. Increase Fiber Intake:

Fiber is beneficial for managing diabetes as it helps regulate blood sugar levels, improves digestive health, and promotes satiety. Include high-fiber foods in your shopping list, such as fresh fruits, vegetables, whole grains, nuts, and seeds. Aim for at least 25-30 grams of fiber daily.

4. Prioritize Lean Proteins:
Choose lean protein sources to support muscle health and stabilize blood sugar levels. Include skinless poultry, fish, lean beef, tofu, eggs, and low-fat dairy products. Avoid processed meats, which may contain additives and are often high in sodium and unhealthy fats.

5. Focus on Healthy Fats:
Monounsaturated and polyunsaturated fats are heart-healthy options that can benefit individuals with diabetes.

Incorporate sources like avocados, nuts, seeds, olive oil, and fatty fish (salmon, mackerel, sardines). Limit saturated fats and avoid trans fats found in processed snacks and fried foods.

6. Read Nutritional Labels:

Learn to read and understand food labels on packaged products. Pay attention to total carbohydrate content, including any added sugars or artificial sweeteners. Be aware of portion sizes and aim for controlled carbohydrate intake in each meal. Choose foods with no added sugars, low sodium, and minimal saturated fats.

7. Shop the Perimeter:

The perimeter of the grocery store often houses the fresh produce, dairy, and lean protein sections. Focus on these healthier options and limit the central aisles that tend to contain processed, sugary, and overly packaged foods.

8. Purchase Fresh Produce:

Consume a wide range of vibrant fruits and vegetable. These nutrient-dense foods are low in calories and rich in vitamins, minerals, and fiber. Opt for non-starchy vegetables like spinach, broccoli, cucumbers, peppers, and zucchini. Limit or moderate starchy vegetables like potatoes and corn.

9. Be Cautious with Snack Choices:

Choose healthy snack options like raw nuts, seeds, Greek yogurt, fresh fruit, or veggie sticks. Avoid sugary snacks, sodas, baked goods, and processed snacks that can cause blood sugar spikes.

10. Stay Hydrated:

Don't forget to stock up on water and unsweetened beverages. Limit your intake of sugary drinks, including fruit juices and soda, which can rapidly increase blood sugar levels.

Conclusion:

Managing diabetes begins with smart grocery shopping choices. By planning ahead, focusing on healthy carbohydrates, incorporating fiber and lean proteins, and reading food labels, you can create a diabetes-friendly shopping list. Prioritize fresh produce, healthy fats, and hydration to maintain stable blood sugar levels and promote overall well-being. Remember, a well-balanced diet combined with regular physical activity forms the foundation for successfully managing diabetes.

Reading Food Labels and Understanding Ingredients

Reading food labels and understanding ingredients is a crucial skill in making informed and healthy food choices. Food labels provide valuable information about the nutritional content, portion sizes, and ingredients used in packaged products. This comprehensive note aims to guide you in deciphering food labels and understanding the significance of ingredients, empowering you to make healthier and more conscious food decisions.

1. Serving Size and Servings per Container:
Start by examining the serving size and the number of servings per container. All nutritional information on the label is

based on these serving sizes. Pay attention to portion sizes to accurately track your nutritional intake.

2. Identify Key Nutrients:

Scan the label for essential details regarding nutrients. Look for information on calories, total fat, saturated fat, trans fat, cholesterol, sodium, total carbohydrates, dietary fiber, sugars, and protein. These values provide insight into the nutritional content and can help you manage your intake according to your dietary needs.

3. Calculate Percent Daily Value (%DV):

The %DV helps you understand how a serving of the particular food contributes to your daily nutritional goals based on a 2,000-calorie diet. Aim to choose foods with lower percentages of saturated fat, sodium, and added sugars. Conversely, opt for higher percentages of dietary fiber, vitamins, and minerals.

4. Understand Ingredients:

Familiarize yourself with the ingredient list to gain insights into the composition of the food item. Ingredients are listed in descending order by weight, meaning the first ingredient listed is present in the highest quantity. Pay attention to the following:

a. **Added Sugars:** Look for various forms of added sugars, such as corn syrup, dextrose, cane sugar, or high-fructose corn syrup. Limit foods with high amounts of added sugars, as excessive intake can lead to various health issues.

b. Unhealthy Fats: Identify sources of unhealthy fats like trans fats and high levels of saturated fats. Trans fats should be avoided altogether, while saturated fats should be consumed in moderation.

c. Sodium Content: Monitor the sodium content, especially if you have high blood pressure or are trying to limit your sodium intake. High levels of sodium can contribute to hypertension and other health problems.

d. Allergen Information: Check for allergens such as nuts, gluten, dairy, or soy if you have known allergies or dietary restrictions.

e. Artificial Additives: Steer clear of artificial colors, flavors, preservatives, and sweeteners (like aspartame or saccharin) that can have potential negative health effects.

5. Watch Out for Marketing Claims:

Be cautious of marketing claims on the front of the packaging. Terms like "low fat," "light," or "natural" can be misleading. Verify these claims by examining the nutritional information and ingredient list.

6. Comparing Different Brands:

Take the time to compare similar food products from different brands. Look for options with a lower content of unhealthy ingredients (such as added sugars and saturated fats) and higher amounts of healthy ingredients (such as fiber and protein).

7. Consider Whole Foods:

Whenever possible, choose whole foods over processed or packaged foods. Whole foods, such as fresh fruits, vegetables, lean meats, and whole grains, generally have minimal or no labels at all, promoting a healthier and more natural diet.

Conclusion:

Reading food labels and understanding ingredients is a crucial step in making informed, healthier choices. By paying attention to serving sizes, key nutrients, %DV, and ingredient lists, you can gain a better understanding of the nutritional content and potential health effects of packaged foods. Use this knowledge to select foods that align with your dietary needs and support your overall well-being.

Smart Shopping Strategies for Diabetes-Friendly Foods

For individuals with diabetes, smart shopping strategies are essential to maintain healthy eating habits and manage blood sugar levels. By adopting these strategies, you can make informed choices while grocery shopping, selecting diabetes-friendly foods that are nutritious, low in sugar, and supportive of your overall health. This comprehensive note provides valuable tips and strategies to help you shop smart and prioritize diabetes-friendly foods.

1. Create a Shopping List:
Before heading to the store, plan your meals and snacks for the week. Create a shopping list that includes a variety of diabetes-friendly foods such as whole

grains, lean proteins, fruits, vegetables, and healthy fats. Having a list will keep you focused and reduce the chances of buying unnecessary items.

2. Read Food Labels:

Carefully read food labels to understand the nutritional content of packaged foods. Look for items that are low in added sugars, saturated fats, and sodium. Pay attention to portion sizes and identify foods that provide beneficial nutrients such as fiber, vitamins, and minerals.

3. Choose Complex Carbohydrates:

Rather than simple carbs, choose complex ones that will not spike your blood sugar. These include whole grains like brown rice, quinoa, whole wheat bread, and whole wheat pasta. Complex carbohydrates provide more fiber and nutrients compared to refined carbohydrates, promoting better blood sugar control.

4. Prioritize Fresh Produce:

Load your cart with a variety of fresh fruits and vegetables. These are low in calories, rich in fiber, and packed with vitamins and minerals. Aim for non-starchy vegetables like leafy greens, broccoli, peppers, and cucumbers. Limit starchy vegetables like potatoes and corn, and choose fresh fruits with a lower glycemic index, such as berries and citrus fruits.

5. Include Lean Proteins:

Select lean protein sources that are low in saturated fat and cholesterol. Opt for skinless poultry, fish, lean cuts of meat like turkey or chicken breast, tofu, beans, lentils, and low-fat dairy products. Protein helps maintain muscle health, promotes satiety, and aids in blood sugar control.

6. Incorporate Healthy Fats:

Choose sources of healthy fats, such as avocados, nuts, seeds, olive oil, and fatty fish like salmon, which are rich in omega-3 fatty acids. These fats can improve heart health and help regulate blood sugar levels. Avoid or limit foods high in unhealthy fats, like fried products and processed snacks.

7. Minimize Processed Foods:

Processed foods are often loaded with sodium, bad fats, and hidden sugars. Limit your intake of packaged snacks, sugary beverages, processed meats, and pre-packaged meals. Instead, prioritize whole, unprocessed foods that are closer to their natural state.

8. Stock Up on Healthy Snacks:

Choose nutritious, diabetes-friendly snacks to keep you satiated between meals. Opt for fresh fruits, raw nuts and seeds, Greek yogurt, vegetables with hummus, or homemade protein bars and energy balls. Avoid sugary snacks, baked goods, and processed chips and cookies.

9. Don't Shop Hungry:

Avoid grocery shopping on an empty stomach as it can lead to impulsive purchases and temptations for unhealthy foods. Eat a balanced meal or snack before heading to the store to help you make more mindful choices.

10. Shop the Perimeter:

The perimeter of the grocery store generally contains the freshest and least processed foods, such as produce, lean meats, and dairy products. Focus your shopping on these areas, reducing exposure to processed and sugary items found in the central aisles.

Conclusion:

Using smart shopping strategies is essential for individuals with diabetes to maintain a healthy and balanced diet. By creating a shopping list, reading food labels, choosing complex carbohydrates, prioritizing fresh produce, including lean proteins, opting for healthy fats, minimizing processed foods, and stocking up on nutritious snacks, you can make informed choices and support your diabetes management goals. Remember, a well-planned and diabetes-friendly shopping trip sets the foundation for a healthy lifestyle.

Planning a Diabetic-Friendly Grocery List

When living with diabetes, planning a diabetic-friendly grocery list is an essential step towards maintaining a healthy lifestyle. By selecting nutritious and balanced foods, you can effectively manage blood sugar levels and support overall well-being. This comprehensive note provides valuable tips for planning a diabetic-friendly grocery list that includes a variety of healthy options while avoiding foods that can negatively impact blood sugar control.

1. Seek advice from a qualified dietitian or healthcare professional:
Before creating your grocery list, consider consulting a healthcare professional or registered dietitian who specializes in

diabetes management. They can provide personalized guidance based on your specific needs, recommend portion sizes, and address any dietary restrictions you may have.

2. Prioritize Whole Foods:

Aim to make the majority of your grocery list consist of whole foods, as they are generally more nutritious and have a milder impact on blood sugar levels. Include items such as fresh fruits, vegetables, lean proteins, whole grains, and healthy fats in their natural forms.

3. Focus on High-Fiber Foods:

Choose foods that are rich in dietary fiber as they can help regulate blood sugar levels and promote healthy digestion. Include items like whole grain bread, brown rice, quinoa, oats, legumes (beans, lentils, chickpeas), fruits, and vegetables in your grocery list.

4. Select Lean Proteins:

Opt for lean protein sources that are low in saturated fats and beneficial for maintaining a balanced diet. Include skinless poultry, fish (salmon, tuna, trout), eggs, low-fat dairy products (yogurt, cottage cheese), tofu, and legumes in your grocery list.

5. Include Healthy Fats:

Don't forget to incorporate healthy fats into your grocery list. Choose sources like avocados, nuts (almonds, walnuts, pistachios), seeds (chia seeds, flaxseeds, pumpkin seeds), olive oil, and fatty fish (salmon, mackerel, sardines). These fats can provide essential nutrients and promote heart health.

6. Limit Added Sugars:

Read food labels carefully and avoid products with high amounts of added sugars. Look for terms like sucrose, high-fructose corn syrup, maltose, and other sweeteners, and minimize the consumption of sugary snacks, desserts, and sugary beverages.

7. Include Low-Glycemic Index Foods:
Consider including low-glycemic index (GI) foods in your grocery list. These foods release glucose gradually into the bloodstream, helping to stabilize blood sugar levels. Examples of low-GI foods include whole grains, certain fruits (apples, berries), non-starchy vegetables, and legumes.

8. Choose Low-Sodium Options:
Limit your intake of sodium to help manage blood pressure and reduce the risk of cardiovascular issues. Opt for low-sodium or no-salt-added versions of canned foods, sauces, and condiments. Instead of using a lot of salt to season your

food, use herbs, spices, and natural flavorings.

9. Plan for Balanced Meals:

Ensure your grocery list supports balanced meals. Consider planning for appropriate portion sizes of carbohydrates, proteins, and fats in each meal. Include a variety of colorful fruits and vegetables, whole grains, lean proteins, and healthy fats to create well-rounded and satisfying meals.

10. Don't Forget Hydration:

Include water and unsweetened beverages on your grocery list. In order to stay hydrated and preserve general health, water is necessary. Limit your intake of sugary drinks and fruit juices, which can cause blood sugar spikes.

Conclusion:

Planning a diabetic-friendly grocery list is a key step towards managing and controlling diabetes effectively. By prioritizing whole foods, high-fiber options, lean proteins, healthy fats, and low-sodium choices while limiting added sugars, you can create a well-balanced and nutritious meal plan. Personalize your grocery list according to your specific dietary needs and consult with healthcare professionals for individualized guidance. Remember, a diabetic-friendly grocery list sets the foundation for a healthy eating pattern that supports optimal blood sugar control and overall well-being.

Chapter 11. Managing Special Occasions with Diabetes

Special occasions such as birthdays, weddings, holiday parties, and other celebrations can often pose challenges for individuals with diabetes. However, with proper planning and proactive management, it is possible to enjoy these events while still maintaining good blood sugar control. Here are some comprehensive tips for managing special occasions with diabetes:

1. **Plan ahead**: Before the event, make sure to discuss your dietary needs with the event organizer or host, especially if the occasion involves serving a meal. Request that diabetic-friendly options be made

available, and inform them about your specific dietary restrictions.

2. Monitor blood sugar levels: Regularly monitor your blood sugar levels leading up to and during the event. This will allow you to adjust your treatment plan accordingly and prevent any unexpected spikes or drops in blood sugar levels.

3. Stay active: Engage in physical activity before or after the event. Exercise helps regulate blood sugar levels and can offset any indulgences during the celebration. Consider taking a brisk walk, dancing, or participating in other enjoyable physical activities.

4. Opt for healthier food choices: When it comes to food, be mindful of your choices. Fill your plate with vegetables, lean proteins, and whole grains, and limit your intake of sugary and high-carbohydrate foods. Savor your chosen treats in moderation, and practice portion control.

5. Alcohol consumption: If you choose to drink alcohol, do so in moderation and be aware of its impact on blood sugar levels. Alcohol can cause delayed hypoglycemia, so it's important to monitor your blood sugar levels closely. Avoid sugary mixed drinks and opt for light beer or dry wines instead.

6. Carry emergency snacks: Always have a source of fast-acting carbohydrates on hand, such as glucose tablets or juice, in case of low blood sugar (hypoglycemia) emergencies. This will ensure you can quickly address any unexpected drops in your blood sugar levels.

7. Stay hydrated: Drink plenty of water throughout the event to stay hydrated and help regulate blood sugar levels. Avoid sugary drinks, as they can cause rapid spikes in blood sugar.

8. Communicate with family and friends: Inform your close family and friends about your diabetes and educate them on the signs and symptoms of low or high blood sugar. This will ensure that they can provide assistance if needed and support your efforts to manage your blood sugar levels during the event.

9. Pack necessary supplies: Before attending the special occasion, double-check that you have all the necessary diabetes supplies, including insulin, glucometer, test strips, and extra batteries if using an insulin pump. Always carry them with you in case you need to monitor your blood sugar levels or administer insulin.

10. Stress management: Special occasions can sometimes be stressful, and stress can impact blood sugar levels. Practice stress-management techniques like deep breathing, mindfulness exercises, or engaging in a calming hobby to help mitigate any stress and maintain stable blood sugar levels.

Remember, it is essential to consult with your healthcare team for personalized advice and guidance specific to your needs. With proper planning, awareness, and self-care, you can successfully navigate special occasions while effectively managing your diabetes.

Navigating Holiday and Festive Meals

Holiday and festive meals are often filled with indulgent and calorie-dense dishes, which can pose challenges for individuals trying to maintain a healthy lifestyle or manage specific dietary needs. However, with mindful planning and some strategies in place, it is possible to enjoy these meals while still making healthy choices. Here are some comprehensive tips for navigating holiday and festive meals:

1. Be mindful of portion sizes: It's easy to overindulge during holiday meals, leading to excess calorie intake. Be mindful of your portion sizes and aim to fill your plate with a balance of healthy options. Begin with smaller servings and enjoy every taste. Allow yourself to enjoy your favorite dishes while practicing moderation.

2. Prioritize vegetables and salads: Incorporate a variety of vegetables and salads into your meal. These nutrient-dense options will provide essential vitamins, minerals, and dietary fiber while keeping calorie intake in check. Try to load your plate with as many vegetables as possible.

3. Choose lean protein: Opt for lean protein sources such as turkey, chicken, fish, or legumes. They are lower in fat and calories compared to heavier protein options. Protein helps keep you feeling full and satisfied, which can deter you from overindulging in unhealthy choices.

4. Be cautious with sauces and dressings: Sauces, gravies, and dressings can be high in added sugars, unhealthy fats, and sodium. Use them sparingly and opt for lighter options when available. Consider using herbs, spices, and citrus juices to flavor your dishes instead.

5. Limit sugary beverages: Be cautious of sugary drinks such as fruit punches, sodas, and holiday cocktails. They can contribute to excess calorie intake and cause blood sugar spikes. Opt for water, unsweetened teas, or diluted fruit juices instead.

6. Watch out for high-fat and fried foods: Be mindful of foods that are high in unhealthy fats, such as deep-fried dishes and dishes prepared with excessive amounts of butter or oil. These can lead to increased cholesterol levels and weight gain. Instead, opt for baked, roasted, or grilled foods.

7. Plan ahead and bring a healthy option: If you are attending a potluck-style gathering or a meal at someone else's home, offer to bring a healthy dish or side. This allows you to have a healthy option on the table and ensures you have something nutritious to fill your plate with.

8. Enjoy mindfully: Slow down and savor each bite. Eating mindfully allows you to fully enjoy the flavors of the meal and recognize when you are satisfied, preventing overeating. Pace your eating by setting down your utensils and conversing between bites.

9. Stay active: Incorporate physical activity into your day, either before or after the festive meal. Physical activity can help balance blood sugar levels, burn calories, and promote a sense of well-being.

10. Manage stress: The holiday season can be stressful, and stress can lead to emotional eating or unhealthy food choices. To reduce stress, try stress-reduction methods like deep breathing, meditation, or doing things you enjoy.

Remember, it's essential to listen to your body and make choices that align with your specific dietary needs and health goals. By being mindful, practicing moderation, and incorporating healthier options, you can navigate holiday and festive meals while still enjoying the spirit of the season.

Strategies for Handling Food Temptations and Social Pressure

Food temptations and social pressure can make it challenging to stick to a healthy eating plan or dietary restrictions. However, with some strategies in place, it is possible to navigate these situations and make choices that align with your goals. Here are some comprehensive tips for handling food temptations and social pressure:

1. Set clear goals and priorities: Establish your health goals and priorities, and remind yourself of them regularly. This will help you stay focused and motivated when faced with food temptations or social pressure.

2. Be prepared: Plan your meals and snacks in advance, and have healthy options readily available. If you have a specific dietary restriction, ensure you have suitable alternatives on hand. By having nutritious options available, you'll be less likely to give in to temptations.

3. Practice portion control: If you're faced with a tempting food, consider enjoying a smaller portion rather than completely avoiding it. Allow yourself a taste or a small serving, savoring the flavor without overindulging. Moderation is key.

4. Focus on healthier alternatives: If there are healthier alternatives available, choose those options instead. Look for dishes that are lower in added sugars, unhealthy fats, or refined carbohydrates. For example, opt for fresh fruit instead of sugary desserts or choose whole grain options over refined grains.

5. Utilize distraction techniques: Engage in activities or conversations that divert your attention away from food. Socialize with friends or family, participate in games or activities, or involve yourself in conversations away from the food table. This reduces the likelihood of mindless grazing or overeating.

6. Communicate your dietary needs: If you have dietary restrictions, communicate them to your friends, family, and hosts. Let them know about your specific needs and restrictions, so they can better understand and support your choices.

7. Offer to bring a dish: When attending a social gathering or event, offer to bring a dish that aligns with your dietary needs. This ensures that there will be at least one option available that you can enjoy while also sharing with others.

8. Be assertive yet polite: If you're feeling pressured to indulge in food that doesn't align with your goals or needs, politely and assertively decline. You can simply say, "No, thank you" or offer an explanation about your dietary restrictions, depending on the situation. Never forget that putting your health and wellbeing first is acceptable.

9. Seek support: Surround yourself with supportive individuals who understand and respect your dietary choices. Share your goals and challenges with them, and lean on their encouragement and understanding during social gatherings. Having a support system can make it easier to resist temptations and navigate social pressure.

10. Practice self-compassion: If you do have an occasional indulgence or give in to social pressure, be kind to yourself. Avoid feelings of guilt or shame. Acknowledge that it's a part of the journey, and get back on track with your healthy eating plan as soon as possible. Recall that consistency holds greater significance than perfection.

By implementing these strategies, you can effectively navigate food temptations and social pressure, making choices that align with your goals and dietary needs. Stay focused, be prepared, and remember to prioritize your health and well-being.

Chapter 12. Incorporating Physical Activity into Diabetes Management

Regular physical activity is an essential component of diabetes management. It can help improve insulin sensitivity, regulate blood sugar levels, manage weight, lower cardiovascular risk, and enhance overall well-being. If you have diabetes, here are some comprehensive tips on incorporating physical activity into your routine:

1. Consult with your healthcare team: Before starting any exercise regimen, consult with your healthcare team, especially if you have any diabetes-related complications. They can provide tailored advice, recommend appropriate activities, and ensure your safety while exercising.

2. Select enjoyable activities: Look for physical pursuits that you actually enjoy. This makes it more likely that you will stay with them in the long run. Whether it's walking, swimming, dancing, cycling, or engaging in team sports, select activities that bring you satisfaction and make you more motivated to be active.

3. Aim for a combination of aerobic and strength training exercises: Incorporate a variety of exercises into your routine to experience maximum benefits. Aerobic activities like brisk walking, jogging, or cycling help improve cardiovascular health, while strength training exercises such as weightlifting or resistance training help build muscle mass and improve glucose metabolism.

4. Start slowly and gradually increase intensity: If you're new to physical activity, start with low-impact exercises and gradually increase the intensity and duration over time. This lowers the chance of injury and enables your body to adjust. Follow the "talk test" - if you can comfortably carry a conversation during exercise, you're at a suitable intensity.

5. Monitor blood sugar levels: Regularly monitor your blood sugar levels before, during, and after exercise, especially if you take insulin or medications that can cause hypoglycemia (low blood sugar). This helps you understand how your body responds to physical activity and make any necessary adjustments to your treatment plan.

6. Stay hydrated: Drink plenty of water before, during, and after exercise to prevent dehydration. Proper hydration supports optimal blood sugar regulation and overall performance during physical activity.

7. Schedule exercise: Treat physical activity as an important appointment in your daily routine. Set specific times for exercise and make it a priority. Consistency is key to reaping the benefits of regular physical activity.

8. Find opportunities to be active throughout the day: Look for ways to incorporate physical activity into your daily life. Use the stairs rather than the elevator, go nearby on foot or by bicycle, or take up an active hobby like dancing or gardening. These small bursts of activity can add up and contribute to your overall fitness level.

9. Consider exercising with a partner or joining a class: Finding a workout partner or joining exercise classes or groups can provide accountability, motivation, and social support. Additionally, it can add fun and enjoyment to exercise.

10. Listen to your body: Pay attention to how your body feels during and after exercise. If you experience any unusual symptoms like dizziness, chest pain, or extreme fatigue, consult your healthcare team. Adjust your routine as needed to ensure your safety and well-being.

Incorporating physical activity into your diabetes management can have numerous benefits for your overall health. Remember to start slowly, be consistent, and personalize your exercise routine based on your preferences and abilities. With time, regular physical activity will become a natural and rewarding part of your diabetes care

Benefits of Exercise for Diabetes

Frequent exercise is essential for managing diabetes. Whether you have type 1 or type 2 diabetes, engaging in physical activity offers numerous benefits that can help improve your overall health and control blood sugar levels. In this note, we will explore the key advantages of exercise for individuals with diabetes.

1. Improved Blood Sugar Control:

Regular exercise helps your body utilize insulin more effectively, resulting in better blood sugar (glucose) control. Physical activity encourages muscle cells to take up more glucose from the bloodstream, reducing the amount of glucose circulating in your system. This leads to fewer spikes and more stable blood sugar levels, reducing the risk of complications associated with diabetes.

2. Weight Management:

Exercise is an essential component of weight management, and maintaining a healthy weight is key for managing type 2 diabetes. Engaging in physical activity can help you burn calories, reduce body fat, and maintain muscle mass. By achieving and maintaining a healthy weight, you can significantly enhance insulin sensitivity and improve overall blood sugar control.

3. Increased Insulin Sensitivity:

Regular exercise enhances the body's sensitivity to insulin, allowing cells to utilize glucose more efficiently. Improved insulin sensitivity means your body requires less insulin to transport glucose from the bloodstream to the cells. This can be particularly beneficial for individuals with insulin resistance commonly seen in type 2 diabetes.

4. Cardiovascular Health:

Diabetes is associated with a higher risk of cardiovascular conditions such as heart disease, high blood pressure, and stroke. Regular exercise helps reduce these risks by improving cardiovascular health. Exercise strengthens the heart, improves blood circulation, and lowers blood pressure and bad cholesterol levels (LDL), decreasing the likelihood of experiencing cardiovascular complications.

5. Stress Reduction:

Stress can have a detrimental effect on blood sugar levels, and having diabetes can make life stressful. Exercise is an effective stress-reducing strategy that triggers the release of endorphins, which are natural mood boosters. By participating in physical activity, you can alleviate stress, anxiety, and depression associated with diabetes management, leading to improved mental well-being.

6. Increased Energy and Improved Sleep:

Exercise increases energy levels by improving muscle strength and endurance, allowing individuals with diabetes to perform daily activities more efficiently. Furthermore, regular physical activity promotes better sleep quality, which is essential for overall health and diabetes management. A good night's sleep can positively influence insulin sensitivity and blood sugar control.

7. Reduced Risk of Complications:
Consistent exercise can help reduce the risks of long-term complications associated with diabetes. These complications include cardiovascular diseases, nerve damage (neuropathy), kidney disease (nephropathy), eye problems (retinopathy), and foot complications. By engaging in exercise, you improve blood flow, lower cholesterol levels, and enhance overall health, mitigating the likelihood of developing these complications.

Conclusion:
In conclusion, exercise offers numerous advantages for individuals with diabetes, regardless of the type. By incorporating

regular physical activity into your routine, you can improve blood sugar control, manage weight, increase insulin sensitivity, enhance cardiovascular health, reduce stress, boost energy levels, and minimize the risk of long-term complications. It is essential, however, to consult with your healthcare provider before starting any exercise program to ensure it aligns with your specific needs and medical considerations.

Tailoring an Exercise Plan to Fit Individual Needs

As a diabetes patient, it is important to understand that exercise plays a vital role in managing your condition. Regular physical activity can help control blood sugar levels, improve insulin sensitivity, lower the risk of cardiovascular diseases, and enhance overall well-being. However, it is crucial to tailor your exercise plan to meet your specific needs as an individual with diabetes. Here are some key considerations to keep in mind when developing an exercise plan:

1. **Consult with your healthcare team**: Before starting an exercise routine, seek guidance from your healthcare team, including your doctor and a registered dietitian or diabetes educator. They can provide valuable insights based on your medical history, current health status, and any specific considerations related to your diabetes.

2. **Establish realistic goals**: Work with your healthcare team to set realistic and attainable fitness goals. These objectives have to be SMART—specific, measurable, realistic, relevant, and time-bound.

Examples may include improving blood sugar control, losing weight, increasing physical endurance, or improving overall fitness.

3. Choose the right type of exercise: Aim for a combination of aerobic exercises (such as walking, swimming, cycling), strength training (using weights or resistance bands), and flexibility exercises (such as yoga or stretching). Each type of exercise offers unique benefits for diabetes management, so it's important to include a variety of activities in your routine.

4. Monitor glucose levels: Regularly check your blood glucose levels before, during, and after exercise to understand how different activities affect your body. This will help you determine if you need to adjust your medication dosage, food intake, or exercise intensity and duration.

5. Time your exercise with medication and meals: Coordinate your exercise sessions with your medication schedule and meals to avoid potential fluctuations in blood sugar levels. Depending on your unique needs, it may be helpful to consume a small snack before exercise or adjust medication timing under the guidance of your healthcare team.

6. Stay hydrated: Maintain proper hydration by drinking water before, during, and after exercise. Dehydration can impact blood sugar levels and overall exercise performance, so it is essential to prioritize hydration throughout your workout.

7. Don't forget warm-ups and cool-downs: Prioritize warm-up exercises (such as light cardio and stretching) before starting any vigorous activity. Your body gets ready for exercise and injuries are avoided as a result. Similarly, cool-down exercises (such as gentle stretching) after workouts can promote recovery and prevent dizziness or blood pressure fluctuations.

8. Listen to your body: Pay attention to any signs or symptoms that may indicate fluctuations in blood sugar levels, such as dizziness, shakiness, or rapid heartbeat. Check your blood sugar levels and cease exercising if you encounter any of these symptoms. Adjust your treatment accordingly and consult your healthcare team if necessary.

9. Track your progress: Keep a record of your exercise activities, blood sugar levels, and any adjustments you make to your medication or food intake. This will help you understand what works best for your body and enable you to make informed decisions regarding your exercise routine.

10. Continuously re-evaluate and adapt: As your fitness level improves and your overall health changes, work with your healthcare team to regularly review and adjust your exercise plan accordingly. Periodically reassess your goals, modify your routine, and stay committed to a lifelong habit of physical activity.

Remember, the best exercise plan is one that fits your individual needs as a diabetes patient. By working with your healthcare team, staying consistent, and making exercise a priority in your daily routine, you can effectively manage your diabetes while improving your overall health and well-being.

Combining Exercise and Meal Planning

Combining exercise with meal planning is essential for managing diabetes effectively. Regular physical activity helps control blood sugar levels, increases insulin sensitivity, and improves overall health. At the same time, a well-balanced meal plan ensures that you consume the right nutrients to support your exercise routine and maintain stable blood sugar levels. Here are some key considerations for combining exercise and meal planning as a diabetes patient:

1. **Consult your healthcare team**: Before starting any exercise program or making significant changes to your meal plan, consult with your healthcare team, including your doctor and a registered dietitian or diabetes educator. They can

provide personalized guidance based on your medical history, current health status, and specific requirements related to your diabetes management.

2. Set realistic goals: Establish realistic goals that align with your diabetes management and overall health. Work with your healthcare team to define goals such as improving blood sugar control, losing weight, increasing physical fitness, or managing other cardiovascular risk factors.

3. Choose the right exercises: Aim for a combination of aerobic exercises (e.g., walking, cycling, swimming), strength training, and flexibility exercises. Aerobic exercises help improve cardiovascular health and can lower blood sugar levels, while strength training can increase muscle mass and improve insulin sensitivity. Flexibility exercises such as yoga or stretching improve mobility and help prevent injuries.

4. Consider timing and intensity: Plan the timing and duration of your exercise sessions in coordination with your meal plan and medication schedule. Depending on your unique needs, exercising before or after meals may help manage blood sugar levels. Start with low-to-moderate-intensity workouts and gradually increase intensity and duration as advised by your healthcare team.

5. Monitor blood sugar levels: Regularly check your blood sugar levels before, during, and after exercise to understand how different activities and meal plans impact your body. This knowledge will help you make necessary adjustments to your routine, meals, or medication to maintain stable blood sugar levels.

6. Fuel your body with balanced meals: Focus on a balanced meal plan that includes a mix of carbohydrates, proteins, and healthy fats. Choose complex carbohydrates such as whole grains, legumes, and vegetables, as they have a steadier impact on blood sugar levels. Include lean proteins and healthy fats to promote satiety and provide sustained energy.

7. Portion control: Be mindful of portion sizes and aim for consistent carbohydrate intake throughout the day. Consult with a registered dietitian to learn appropriate portion sizes and to design a meal plan that meets your specific needs.

8. Hydration: Stay adequately hydrated by drinking plenty of water throughout the day, before, during, and after exercise. Avoid sugary drinks and be cautious of excessive fluid intake if you have any kidney-related complications.

9. Plan for special occasions: Plan ahead for special occasions or events that involve different meal options or intense physical activity. Discuss with your healthcare team how to adjust your meal plan and medication to maintain blood sugar control during these situations.

10. Regular monitoring and adjustments: Keep a record of your exercise routine, meals, and blood sugar levels. Regularly review and analyze this data to identify patterns and make necessary adjustments to your exercise and meal plan in consultation with your healthcare team.

By combining exercise with a well-planned meal routine, you can effectively manage your diabetes. Working closely with your healthcare team, monitoring your blood sugar levels, and making informed choices regarding exercise and meals will help you control blood sugar, improve overall health, and reduce the risk of complications associated with diabetes. Remember, consistency and ongoing communication with your healthcare team are key to achieving long-term success in managing diabetes through exercise and meal planning.

Chapter 13. Tracking Progress and Adjusting Meal Plan

Tracking your progress and making adjustments to your meal plan are important aspects of effectively managing diabetes. By monitoring your blood sugar levels, observing your body's response to different foods, and regularly reviewing your meal plan, you can make informed decisions to maintain stable blood sugar levels and optimize your overall health. Here are some key considerations for tracking progress and adjusting your meal plan:

1. **Blood sugar monitoring**: Regularly check your blood sugar levels as advised by your healthcare team. Tracking your blood sugar levels before and after meals,

as well as before and after physical activity, can help you understand how different foods and exercises affect your body. This information will assist you in making appropriate adjustments to your meal plan.

2. Keep a food diary: Maintain a food diary to track your daily dietary intake. Record the types and amounts of food you consume, along with the time and your corresponding blood sugar levels. This diary will help you identify patterns and recognize the impact of different foods on your blood sugar levels.

3. Monitor portion sizes: Pay close attention to portion sizes and measure your food accurately. Using measuring cups, a food scale, or visual references can help you maintain consistent carbohydrate intake and avoid blood sugar fluctuations. Consult with a registered dietitian to understand appropriate portion sizes for optimal diabetes management.

4. Carbohydrate counting: Learn to count carbohydrates in your meals. This method involves calculating the total grams of carbohydrates consumed and matching it with the appropriate insulin dosage or medications. Carbohydrate counting can provide more precise control over blood sugar levels and help you adjust your meal plan accordingly.

5. Glycemic index awareness: Become familiar with the glycemic index (GI) of different foods. Based on how they affect blood sugar levels, carbohydrates are ranked on the GI. Foods with low GI values, such as whole grains, legumes, and non-starchy vegetables, tend to cause a slower and more stable rise in blood sugar levels. Incorporating more low GI foods into your meal plan can be beneficial for blood sugar control.

6. Work with a registered dietitian: Collaborate with a registered dietitian who specializes in diabetes management. They can review your food diary, blood sugar readings, and overall progress, and provide personalized recommendations to adjust your meal plan. A dietitian can also assist in fine-tuning your carbohydrate counting, glycemic index knowledge, and portion control.

7. Adapt your meal plan: Based on the information gathered through blood sugar monitoring and food tracking, make appropriate adjustments to your meal plan. This may involve modifying the types and quantities of carbohydrates, distributing carbohydrate intake throughout the day, adjusting protein and fat intake, or refining meal timings to maintain stable blood sugar levels.

8. Regular reviews and assessments: Schedule regular follow-ups with your healthcare team to review your progress, discuss any challenges, and make adjustments to your meal plan or medication regimen as needed. Monitoring your progress and working closely with your healthcare team will help ensure ongoing success in managing diabetes.

9. Lifestyle changes: Recognize that factors beyond food and exercise can influence blood sugar control. Stress, sleep, medication changes, and other lifestyle factors can have an impact. Track these factors along with your meal plan and blood sugar levels to identify potential correlations and make appropriate adjustments.

10. Stay motivated: Managing diabetes requires lifelong commitment and persistence. Stay motivated by focusing on the positive changes you observe in your blood sugar levels, overall health, and well-being. Celebrate your achievements and seek support from healthcare professionals, support groups, or loved ones to maintain your dedication to managing diabetes.

By actively monitoring your progress, adjusting your meal plan, and collaborating with your healthcare team, you can effectively manage your diabetes and maintain stable blood sugar levels. Remember, individual responses may vary, so it's important to personalize your meal plan according to your specific needs and consult with your healthcare team for expert guidance throughout your journey.

Importance of Regular Blood Sugar Monitoring

Regular blood sugar monitoring plays a vital role in managing diabetes effectively. Monitoring your blood sugar levels allows you to gain insights into how your body is responding to various factors, such as food, exercise, medications, and stress. By closely tracking your blood sugar levels, you can make informed decisions to adjust your treatment plan, maintain stable blood sugar levels, and minimize the risk of complications. Here are key reasons why regular blood sugar monitoring is important:

1. Understanding the impact of food: Monitoring blood sugar levels before and after meals helps you understand how different foods affect your body. By tracking these levels, you can identify which foods cause significant spikes or drops in blood sugar, allowing you to adjust your meal plan accordingly. This knowledge helps maintain stable blood sugar levels and optimizes your overall diabetes management.

2. Assessing medication effectiveness: Regular blood sugar monitoring helps determine how well your current medication or insulin regimen is working. By comparing your blood sugar levels with target ranges, you can evaluate whether your medications require adjustment. This information is crucial for ensuring optimal medication dosages and avoiding complications related to either low or high blood sugar levels.

3. Detecting trends and patterns: Tracking blood sugar levels over a period of time helps identify trends and patterns. This information can reveal how your blood sugar fluctuates throughout the day, allowing you to adjust your meal planning, physical activity, and medication timings accordingly. It also helps identify potential triggers, such as specific foods or stressors, that may impact your blood sugar levels.

4. Preventing hypo- and hyperglycemia: Hypoglycemia (low blood sugar) and hyperglycemia (high blood sugar) can be potentially dangerous conditions for people with diabetes. Regular blood sugar monitoring enables you to detect and address early signs of both hypo- and hyperglycemia promptly. By addressing these imbalances in a timely manner, you can prevent severe complications and maintain stable blood sugar levels.

5. Supporting treatment adjustments: Blood sugar monitoring provides valuable data that healthcare professionals can use to make informed treatment adjustments. In collaboration with your healthcare team, tracking your blood sugar levels allows them to tailor your medication dosages, insulin regimens, and meal plans to meet your specific needs. This personalized approach helps optimize your diabetes management and effectively control blood sugar levels.

6. Promoting proactive self-care: Regular blood sugar monitoring empowers you to take an active role in your diabetes management. By tracking your blood sugar levels, you become more aware of the impact of your lifestyle choices on your health. This awareness motivates you to make informed decisions about your diet, exercise routine, and overall self-care, ultimately improving your diabetes control and well-being.

7. Identifying potential complications: Consistent blood sugar monitoring helps identify potential complications associated with diabetes. Fluctuating blood sugar levels can lead to long-term complications, such as nerve damage, kidney problems, and cardiovascular diseases. Early detection of abnormal blood sugar patterns through monitoring allows for timely intervention and prevention of serious complications.

8. Accountability and motivation: Monitoring your blood sugar levels regularly holds you accountable for your diabetes management. It serves as a reminder to make healthy choices and stick to your treatment plan. Additionally, observing positive changes in your blood sugar levels can be motivating and reinforce the importance of maintaining good diabetes control.

Remember, it is important to work closely with your healthcare team to develop an individualized blood sugar monitoring plan that fits your specific needs. They will guide you on how often to monitor, which blood glucose monitor to use, and what target ranges to aim for. Regular blood sugar monitoring, in combination with a comprehensive diabetes management plan, helps you maintain stable blood sugar levels, reduce the risk of complications, and live a healthy life with diabetes.

Evaluating the Effectiveness of the Meal Plan

Evaluating the effectiveness of your meal plan is crucial for managing diabetes. It allows you to assess how well your current dietary choices and portion sizes are supporting your blood sugar control, weight management, and overall health. By regularly evaluating your meal plan, you can make necessary adjustments to optimize your diabetes management. Here are key considerations for evaluating the effectiveness of your meal plan for diabetes:

1. **Blood sugar control:** Monitoring your blood sugar levels before and after meals is essential in evaluating the effectiveness of your meal plan. Compare your blood sugar readings to target ranges suggested by your healthcare team. Consistently high or low readings may indicate the need for adjustments to your meal plan, such as modifying the types and amounts of carbohydrates, adjusting portion sizes, or altering your eating schedule.

2. Glycemic load: Assess the impact of different foods on your blood sugar by considering their glycemic load. Foods with a high glycemic load cause a more significant rise in blood sugar levels, while those with a low glycemic load result in a slower and more gradual increase. Evaluating the glycemic load of the foods you consume can help you make informed choices to maintain stable blood sugar levels.

3. Weight management: If weight management is a goal, evaluate how your meal plan is supporting your efforts. Regularly monitor your weight and assess if your current meal plan enables you to achieve or maintain a healthy weight. If adjustments are needed, consider working with a registered dietitian who can guide you in making appropriate modifications to your calorie intake, portion sizes, and nutrient distribution.

4. Nutritional balance: Evaluate the nutritional balance of your meal plan by considering essential nutrients like carbohydrates, proteins, fats, vitamins, and minerals. Ensure that your meals provide a variety of nutrient-dense foods that meet your individual requirements. Consult with a registered dietitian to review your meal plan's nutritional composition and make necessary adjustments to ensure adequate intake of key nutrients.

5. Satiety and hunger management: Consider how well your meal plan keeps you feeling satiated and manages hunger. Evaluating these aspects helps ensure that your meal plan provides the necessary energy and nutrients while preventing excessive overeating or periods of prolonged hunger. Adjusting the composition of meals, such as incorporating more fiber-rich foods and proteins, can enhance satiety and maintain stable blood sugar levels throughout the day.

6. Individualized approach: The effectiveness of a meal plan can vary from person to person, considering factors such as personal preferences, cultural influences, lifestyle, and individual response to foods. Evaluate how well your meal plan aligns with your unique needs and preferences. Allow for flexibility in your meal plan to accommodate variations while maintaining consistency in portion sizes, nutrient distribution, and overall carbohydrate control.

7. Collaboration with healthcare team: Regularly consult with your healthcare team, including your doctor and a registered dietitian or diabetes educator, to review the effectiveness of your meal plan. They can provide professional guidance, interpret your blood sugar readings, and help identify potential adjustments to optimize your diabetes management.

8. Long-term sustainability: Assess the long-term sustainability of your meal plan. An effective meal plan should be practical, enjoyable, and fit within your lifestyle. If your current meal plan is too restrictive, causing frustration or feelings of deprivation, it may not be sustainable in the long run. Seek guidance to make modifications that ensure adherence and enjoyment while meeting your diabetes management goals.

Remember, evaluating the effectiveness of your meal plan is an ongoing process. Regular monitoring, blood sugar checks, and collaboration with healthcare professionals are essential. By continuously assessing and making necessary adjustments, you can optimize your meal plan to support blood sugar control, weight management, and overall well-being as you successfully manage diabetes.

Making Necessary Adjustments for Optimal Diabetes Management

Optimal diabetes management requires making necessary adjustments to various aspects of your treatment plan. By continuously assessing your blood sugar levels, medication regimen, meal plan, physical activity, and overall lifestyle, you can identify areas that need improvement and make necessary adjustments. Here are key considerations for making adjustments to achieve optimal diabetes management:

1. **Blood sugar monitoring**: Regularly monitor your blood sugar levels as recommended by your healthcare team. Tracking your blood sugar readings before and after meals, during physical activity, and at different times of the day helps you identify patterns and fluctuations. Based on these insights, you can make informed adjustments to your treatment plan.

2. **Medication regimen**: Evaluate the effectiveness of your medication regimen in achieving target blood sugar levels. If your blood sugar readings consistently fall outside the recommended range, consult with your doctor to discuss potential adjustments to your medication dosage or type. It's important to collaborate with

your healthcare team to ensure safe and effective changes to your medication regimen.

3. Meal planning: Assess the impact of your meal plan on blood sugar control and overall health. Consider the types and quantities of carbohydrates, proteins, fats, and fiber in your meals. Evaluate the glycemic load of the foods you consume and adjust accordingly. Work with a registered dietitian to make necessary modifications to your meal plan, such as adjusting portion sizes, altering nutrient distribution, or incorporating new healthy choices.

4. Physical activity: Evaluate the role of physical activity in your diabetes management. Assess the duration, intensity, and frequency of your exercise routine and how it affects your blood sugar levels. Based on your findings, make adjustments to your physical activity plan, such as increasing or reducing intensity, modifying exercise duration or timing, or incorporating different types of workouts.

5. Promptly address fluctuating blood sugar levels: Identify potential triggers for fluctuating blood sugar levels, such as specific foods, stress, illness, or medication changes. If you notice consistent patterns, make the necessary adjustments. For example, if certain foods consistently cause elevated blood sugar, consider reducing their consumption or finding alternatives. If stress impacts your blood sugar control, incorporate stress management techniques into your routine, such as mindfulness, relaxation exercises, or seeking support from a mental health professional.

6. Collaborate with your healthcare team: Regularly consult with your healthcare team, including your doctor, registered dietitian, and diabetes educator. Share your blood sugar readings, meal plan, physical activity data, and any other relevant information. Collaborating with your healthcare team ensures that adjustments are made under their guidance, expertise, and supervision.

7. **Educate yourself**: Stay informed about the latest developments in diabetes management and treatments. Attend educational sessions, workshops, or webinars related to diabetes. Read credible sources, such as medical journals or trusted websites, to deepen your knowledge. This knowledge will empower you to actively participate in decisions regarding your treatment plan and make informed adjustments.

8. **Monitor overall health**: Recognize that diabetes management extends beyond

blood sugar control. Regularly monitor and manage other aspects of your health, such as blood pressure, cholesterol levels, and weight. Seek comprehensive care to address any comorbidities or complications associated with diabetes.

9. **Self-reflection and motivation**: Regularly reflect on your progress and set realistic goals for your diabetes management. Celebrate your achievements, no matter how small, and reinforce positive changes in your health and well-being. Stay motivated by connecting with support groups, seeking encouragement from loved ones, or leveraging diabetes management apps and tools.

10. **Long-term planning**: Diabetes management is a lifelong journey. Plan for long-term success by incorporating sustainable lifestyle changes. Avoid fad

diets or temporary solutions. Focus on adopting healthy eating habits, regular physical activity, stress management techniques, and maintaining a positive mindset.

Remember, making necessary adjustments for optimal diabetes management requires ongoing assessment, collaboration with your healthcare team, and a commitment to self-care. By proactively identifying areas that need improvement and implementing necessary changes, you can achieve stable blood sugar control, minimize complications, and lead a healthier life with diabetes.

Chapter 14. Conclusion

In conclusion, "The Comprehensive Diabetes Food List and Meal Plan" provides an invaluable resource for individuals with diabetes seeking to effectively manage their condition through proper nutrition. This comprehensive guide offers a wealth of information and practical guidance on creating a balanced meal plan, making appropriate food choices, and understanding the impact of different foods on blood sugar levels.

Throughout the book, readers are equipped with essential tools, including a comprehensive food list categorized by macronutrients and glycemic index. This allows individuals to make informed decisions when selecting foods that align with their dietary needs and diabetes management goals. The meal plans provided in the book offer flexible options with delicious and nutritious recipes that cater to various food preferences and cultural influences.

One of the book's primary strengths is its emphasis on personalized and individualized approaches to diabetes management. It acknowledges that each person's experience with diabetes is unique, and one-size-fits-all solutions are inadequate. By encouraging readers to consult with healthcare professionals, registered dietitians, and diabetes educators, the book promotes a collaborative and individualized approach to meal planning and diabetes management.

"The Comprehensive Diabetes Food List and Meal Plan" goes beyond simply providing a list of foods and meal suggestions. It educates readers on the importance of monitoring blood sugar levels, understanding the glycemic load of foods, and recognizing the impact of lifestyle factors on diabetes control. By empowering readers with knowledge, the book enables them to take an active role in their diabetes management and make necessary adjustments for optimal health outcomes.

Furthermore, the book recognizes the significance of long-term sustainability and adherence to a meal plan. It highlights the importance of flexibility, enjoyment, and practicality in creating a meal plan that individuals can maintain over the long term. By encouraging readers to prioritize balanced nutrition, portion control, and regular physical activity, the book promotes a holistic approach to diabetes management.

In summary, "The Comprehensive Diabetes Food List and Meal Plan" is a comprehensive and practical resource that equips individuals with the knowledge and tools they need to successfully manage diabetes through personalized nutrition. With its emphasis on individualization, awareness, and long-term sustainability, the book serves as a valuable companion for anyone seeking to optimize their diabetes management, improve blood sugar control, and enhance overall well-being.